AMBULATORY HYSTEROSCOPY:

An Evidence-Based Guide to Diagnosis and Therapy in the Outpatient Setting

PY:

...ide to

...in the

...d Gynaecology,

...lford, UK

...ology,
...n, UK

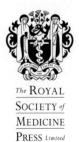

The ROYAL
SOCIETY *of*
MEDICINE
PRESS *Limited*

Published by the Royal Society of Medicine Press Ltd
1 Wimpole Street, London W1G 0AE, UK
Tel: +44 (0)20 7290 2921
Fax: +44 (0)20 7290 2929
Email: publishing@rsm.ac.uk
Website: www.rsmpress.co.uk

British Library Cataloguing in Publication Data
A catalogue record for this book is available from the British Library

ISBN 1-85315-640-X

Distribution in Europe and Rest of World:

Marston Book Services Ltd
PO Box 269
Abingdon
Oxon OX14 4YN, UK
Tel: +44 (0)1235 465500
Fax: +44 (0)1235 465555
Email: direct.order@marston.co.uk

Distribution in the USA and Canada:

Royal Society of Medicine Press Ltd
c/o BookMasters Inc
30 Amberwood Parkway
Ashland, OH 44805, USA
Tel: +1 800 247 6553/+1 800 266 5564
Fax: +1 419 281 6883
Email: order@bookmasters.com

Distribution in Australia and New Zealand:

Elsevier Australia
30-52 Smidmore Street
Marrikville NSW 2204, Australia
Tel: +61 2 9517 8999
Fax: +61 2 9517 2249
Email: service@elsevier.com.au

Editorial services and typesetting by GM & BA Haddock, Ford, Midlothian, UK

Printed by Replika Press Pvt Ltd, India

Contents

Preface

In 1994, the death of the wife of a prominent citizen following an endoscopic procedure prompted her grief-stricken husband to inquire into the experience and qualifications of the performing surgeon resulting in an enquiry. The results of this enquiry were sufficiently disturbing for the UK Royal Colleges of Surgery and of Obstetricians and Gynaecologists to form working parties to generate recommendations for training and accreditation in endoscopy. This work is still in progress. The primary goal of this book is to provide a high-quality text to accompany training, practice and teaching in hysteroscopy. We have made a concentrated effort to compile this text in such a way that it will enhance learning, technical skills, and professional attitudes required to function as a competent hysteroscopist providing specialised ambulatory healthcare to women.

Hysteroscopy has dramatically advanced over the last decade shifting the focus in health-care away from inpatient diagnosis and treatment. Considering the modern equipment and telescopes that are just a few millimetres in diameter, in the hands of a trained operator, out-patient hysteroscopy is possible in most cases. This book will provide guidance on how to set up an outpatient or ambulatory hysteroscopy service and how to write a business case. One of the objectives of performing ambulatory hysteroscopy should be to avoid procedure-related harm to the patient. This book will give an overview of the current risk management strategy for increasing patient safety through ambulatory hysteroscopy.

An Accreditation Council for Gynaecologic Endoscopy was established in 1994 in the US to set criteria for documenting the experience and qualifications of gynaecologists performing advanced endoscopic surgery. In the UK, the Royal Colleges and Universities have developed formal courses and qualifications in hysteroscopy. The European Board and College of Obstetrics and Gynaecology and the European Society of Gynaecological Endoscopy have approved hysteroscopy training programmes which can be adapted, with appropriate adjustments, to suit the overall objectives of the gynaecology training programme in a particular country.

Trainees in a structured educational system will have opportunities for formal instruction, appropriate supervision, critical evaluation and increasing responsibility as they progress. While emphasising traditional approaches to learning, an effort should be made to integrate the latest evidence into a training programme. Learning about hysteroscopy requires acquiring both knowledge and skills. This book provides instructional material on ambulatory diagnostic and operative hysteroscopy. To achieve competence, every trainee should have an individual development and learning plan. There should be a named preceptor who will facilitate training and will help provide a secure, confidential and supportive learning atmosphere for the trainee. Such an environment should enable the trainee to learn the full range of outpatient diagnostic and operative hystero-scopic procedures using this book. This book will compliment the postgraduate special skills modules and training courses in advanced hys-teroscopy which are run by the various colleges and societies for gynaecological endoscopy world-wide.

Senior hysteroscopists running a dedicated clinical service are suitable preceptors for hysteroscopic training of junior doctors and nurses. They will find this text helpful in plan-ning their teaching programmes, which would also be suitable for continuing professional development for established clinicians. During training, we suggest students should have at least one and probably two sessions a week ded-icated to private study using this book . In addi-tion, the knowledge component will be supple-mented by the trainee's attendance at a formal theoretical course, *e.g.* the theory component of the Special Skill Module in Avanced Hystero-scopic Surgery is delivered at the UK Royal College of Obstetricians and Gynaecologists once or twice a year.

This book is written by three experienced clini-cians who are fully conversant with ambulatory hysteroscopy and are teachers in this field. Shagaf Bakour, a Consultant in Obstetrics and Gynaeco-logy and Honorary Senior Lecturer at City Hospital, Birmingham, has completed her Doctor of Medicine in *Evaluation of Ambulatory Diagnosis of Abnormal Uterine Bleeding* and has published wide-ly on the topic. Sian Jones, a Consultant Gynaeco-logist at Bradford Teaching Hospitals NHS Foundation Trust, and Vice President of the British Society for Gynaecological Endoscopy, is a pioneer of nurse hysteroscopy training at Bradford, and National Co-ordinator for National Health Training Courses. Khalid Khan, a Professor of Obstetrics–Gynaecology and Clinical Epidemiology is an Honorary Consultant Gynaecologist at Birming-ham Women's Hospital. He has supervised Doctor of Medicine students in hysteroscopy at the University of Birmingham and is an examiner for the Nurse Hysteroscopy Course at University of Bradford. He has published widely in this field.

We hope you enjoy reading about ambulatory hysteroscopy in the text that follows.

SH Bakour, SE Jones and KS Khan

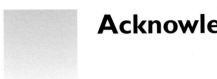

Acknowledgements

No work can ever be completed without the support of many individuals. The authors would like to thank families and friends who supported the writing of this book. We are particularly grateful to the following colleagues and companies for their contributions outlined below:

Mr Linga Dwarakanath MRCOG
Consultant/Honorary Senior Lecturer in Obstetrics and Gynaecology, City Hospital, Birmingham, UK
For providing valuable images for Chapters 2, 4 and 5.

Mr Alaa El-Gobashy MB ChB MSc MD MRCOG
Specialist Registrar, Bradford Royal Infirmary, UK
For providing the text for Chapter 3: Equipment required for ambulatory hysteroscopy.

Mr Joseph Ogah MB BS MRCOG
Specialist Registrar, Bradford Royal Infirmary, UK
For providing the text for Chapter 6: Indications and contra-indications for ambulatory diagnostic hysteroscopy and Chapter 7: Indications for ambulatory operative hysteroscopy.

Dr Janet Wright BSc MB BS MRCOG
Consultant Obstetrician and Gynaecologist and Risk Management Lead, Bradford Royal Infirmary, UK
For providing the text for Chapter 10: Risk management for ambulatory hysteroscopy.

Dr John Chift MB ChB FRCA
Consultant in Anaesthesia and Critical Care Medicine, Lead Obstetric Anaesthetist, City Hospital, Birmingham, UK
For critically reviewing Chapter 5: Pain control in ambulatory hysteroscopy.

Boston Scientific (www.bostonscientific.com)
Boston Scientific Corporate Headquarters,
One Boston Scientific Place, Natick, MA 01760-1537, USA

GyneCare Versapoint® (www.gynecare.com)
GyneCare Division of Ethicon Inc., a Johnson & Johnson Company.
PO Box 151, Somerville, NJ 08876-0151, USA

Karl Storz (www.karlstorz.com)
Karl Storz Media Centre GmbH & Co, Mittelstr. 8, 78532, Tuttlingen, Germany

Microsulis (www.microsulis.co.uk)
Microsulis Medical Ltd, Parklands Business Park, Denmead, Hants, PO7 6XP, UK
For providing the relevant images

1 Introduction

OBJECTIVE : To provide an overview of ambulatory hysteroscopy and how it can best be utilised by readers.

CONTENTS

Historical background
The developing role of hysteroscopy
Structure of the book

Value of the book
Key points

HISTORICAL BACKGROUND

In 1865, Desormeaux developed the first cysto-scope. Before that, Bozzini had performed the first urethroscopy in 1805. Pantaleoni, in 1869, performed the first ambulatory diagnostic and operative hysteroscopy using this instrument to diagnose and treat a haemorrhagic uterine growth with silver nitrate. The modern application of minimally invasive surgery began in the early 1960s when pelviscopy (minimally invasive examination of the pelvic structures) was introduced in Europe and later in the US. Over the next 20 years, endoscopy gained increasing acceptance as a diagnostic tool amongst both gynaecologists and general surgeons. Hystero-scopy was not widely adopted until the advent of cold-light illumination and fibre-optic lenses (see Chapter 3) which improved the image and field of vision for direct endoscopic visualisation of the endometrial cavity. It was Hamou, in 1979, who revolutionised the field of hysteroscopy with new,

improved visual optics and instruments of fine diameter (< 4 mm hysteroscopes). Improved optics, simpler techniques and the ability to perform the examination in conscious patients in the outpatient clinic without the need for cervical dilatation have further popularised hysteroscopy in the 1980s and 1990s. Hysteroscopic procedures, both diagnostic and operative, are now widely used by gynaecologists in the ambulatory setting because of the rapid recovery time, decreased costs and fewer complications.

THE DEVELOPING ROLE OF HYSTEROSCOPY

Healthcare providers are facing increasing demands for improvement in the quality of life of women of all ages. Improvements in service provision are ensured by the active introduction of minimally invasive technologies into all spheres of gynaecological practice. The benefits it provides are extraordinary. The process of positive change towards minimally invasive

Table 1.1 Definitions	
Hysteroscopy	Direct endoscopic visualisation of the endometrial cavity
Cold light	The components of cold light consist of a powerful external light source (halogen or xenon lamps) that is transmitted via a special optical guide into the endometrial cavity with a lens between the light cable and the light box which absorbs the heat before it reaches the patient
Fibre-optic cable/lens	The light-conveying glass fibre that transmits light from the source to the endoscope
Microhysteroscope	A hysteroscope with a fine diameter (2–3 mm)
Minimally invasive surgery	A growing number of surgical procedures that achieve the same surgical result as traditional operations, but are performed with much smaller incisions. This is done with the help of specially designed instruments (endoscopes) which are inserted through small 'keyhole-sized' surgical incisions or through natural orifices for a wide variety of diagnostic and therapeutic interventions
Menorrhagia	A condition of excessive blood loss > 80 ml during menstruation
Dysfunctional uterine bleeding	Heavy or irregular menstrual bleeding that is not caused by an underlying pathological abnormality, such as a fibroid, polyps, or tumours. It is the most common type of abnormal uterine bleeding
Postmenopausal bleeding	Bleeding from the reproductive system that occurs 12 months (6 months in an American definition) or more after cessation of menstrual periods due to menopause

surgery in operative gynaecology is being supported and promoted by the medical community in every possible way.

Hysteroscopy is used extensively in the evaluation of common gynaecological problems, such as premenopausal menstrual disorders and postmenopausal bleeding. It allows direct visualisation of the uterine cavity and the opportunity for targeted biopsy, safe removal of endometrial polyps, treatment of submucus fibroids and adhesions (see Chapters 6 and 7). Diagnostic hysteroscopy has become an important and valuable tool for the gynaecologist in the assessment of many conditions previously evaluated with blind and inaccurate techniques. Terms used in this book are defined in Table 1.1.

Abnormal uterine bleeding is a common presenting symptom in the primary care setting. In women of child-bearing age, a systematic approach to history, physical examination, and laboratory evaluation will enable clinicians to rule out causes such as pregnancy-related disorders, contraception-related bleeding, iatrogenic causes, systemic conditions, and obvious genital tract pathology. Dysfunctional uterine bleeding is diagnosed by exclusion of these causes and accounts for 40% of cases. In women who are at high risk for endometrial cancer, the initial evaluation includes transvaginal ultrasonography, endometrial biopsy, diagnostic hysteroscopy or saline-infusion sonohysterography. This book will illustrate how best to use these tests. For example: women who are at low-risk for endometrial cancer may be assessed initially by transvaginal ultrasonography alone; while women with postmenopausal bleeding may be offered transvaginal ultrasonography with or without hysteroscopy and endometrial biopsy.

Outpatient hysteroscopy has developed into an easy, safe, quick, and effective method of intra-uterine evaluation that provides immediate results, offers the capacity for direct-targeted biopsies of suspicious focal lesions and offers the possibility of immediate treatment of some intra-uterine conditions. It has been facilitated by the availability of small-calibre hysteroscopes. Because of its simplicity and ease, the procedure is in common use for patients with abnormal uterine bleeding or abnormal ultrasound findings and for patients with suspected intra-uterine pathology. The combined procedure – hysteroscopy and endometrial sampling – offers an excellent method to evaluate patients with abnormal uterine bleeding. Transvaginal sonography with or without fluid enhancement complements the uterine evaluation, rather than replacing hysteroscopy. The success of outpatient hysteroscopy depends on the appropriate selection of patients, the absence of contra-indications, adequate instrumentation, meticulous technique and, of course, appropriate training. With this book, readers will be able to make rational clinical decisions about employing hysteroscopic diagnosis and treatment in practice.

STRUCTURE OF THE BOOK

This comprehensive and practical manual covers all important areas of the subject. It is organised in chapters that follow logically and build knowledge about the subject progressively. This book also includes in-depth analysis of outpatient

diagnostic hysteroscopy, the accuracy of diagnostic hysteroscopy, indications for outpatient operative hysteroscopy, its contra-indications, a business case for developing such a service, its risk management, and training and teaching. There are essential key points at the end of each chapter. To enhance learning on the subject, there are questions and answers in the form of Multiple Choice Questions (MCQs) and Objective Structured Clinical Examinations (OSCEs). The answers are provided in a form suitable for feedback at the end of this book.

VALUE OF THE BOOK

This book provides a comprehensive, balanced and pragmatic guide to the entire field of ambulatory hysteroscopy with particular focus on diagnostic and operative techniques. It is an important addition to the literature relating to this extremely exciting and rapidly advancing field of gynaecological practice, which is likely to be applied widely by doctors, nurses and general practitioners. It will complement courses and modules being developed by various specialist societies and postgraduate colleges. Through this book, readers will acquire the knowledge they need to become independent practitioners in hysteroscopy.

This book includes material that has been carefully designed to develop and test the reader's theoretical and practical knowledge of hysteroscopy so as to prompt thought and discussion and thus lead to a better understanding of the subject. Explanatory text is provided throughout and supplemented by key message tables to consolidate study points. Readers will find this book very useful for self-assessment during initial preparation for their examinations as well as final revision. In the continuing education context, the book is ideal as a reference source for qualified doctors and nurses wishing to update themselves with new developments as part of their professional development.

Like medicine generally, hysteroscopy and related healthcare is a rapidly changing field. As developments occur, this text will become out of date. In this book, we have scanned the horizon and provided an overview of current practice. The reader is encouraged to keep up-to-date with the literature for developments in the future.

Key points

➢ Hysteroscopy plays a major role in the rapid diagnosis and treatment of uterine pathology.

➢ Outpatient techniques for hysteroscopic treatment are becoming widely available in hospitals and ambulatory centres.

➢ This book is an evidence-based resource for postgraduate students that will inculcate in-depth learning.

➢ The contents of this book are essential reading for the continuing professional development of doctors and nurses involved in women's health.

➢ This book will provide a step-by-step guide on how to perform hysteroscopy safely and will illustrate how to establish and maintain an ambulatory hysteroscopy service.

2 How to set up an ambulatory (outpatient) service

OBJECTIVE: To familiarise readers with the essential elements for development and delivery of a one-stop ambulatory hysteroscopy service.

CONTENTS

The need for outpatient hysteroscopy
Advantages of a one-stop hysteroscopy clinic
How to set up a one-stop hysteroscopy service

Preparing a business case for a one-stop hysteroscopy clinic
Key points

THE NEED FOR OUTPATIENT HYSTEROSCOPY

It is estimated that more than a quarter of all women will complain of abnormal uterine bleeding (pre- or postmenopausal) at some point during their lives. Abnormal uterine bleeding can have a profound effect on a woman's life. A woman may suffer socially, physically, psychologically and psychosexually. It is important that she gets prompt diagnosis and treatment. The aim of investigations is to exclude endometrial cancer, hyperplasia and benign lesions. Abnormalities are found in about 30% of cases.

Until recently, diagnosis and treatment involved lengthy multiple visits in both primary and secondary care which meant a huge amount of disruption to the patient's life, long waiting times to be seen, and a high rate of major surgery. About 60% of referred women ended up having a hysterectomy and many more had cervical dilatation and uterine curettage under general anaesthesia.

This chapter will provide guidance on outpatient or ambulatory hysteroscopy, a procedure for which inpatient admission and general anaesthesia are not necessary. Considering the modern equipment and telescopes that are just a few millimetres in diameter in the hands of a trained operator, outpatient hysteroscopy is possible in most cases.

In the 1980s, the first one-stop services for abnormal uterine bleeding were started with the pioneering efforts of both gynaecologists and specialist nurses. The development of outpatient hysteroscopy was central to the success of these services. Waiting times were reduced as women were seen in one visit, which included a consultation, ultrasound scan (if appropriate), outpatient hysteroscopy and endometrial sampling leading to an individualised management plan. It has recently become feasible to undertake therapeutic procedures within the same visit.

In the last 10 years, technological improvements have led to the production of smaller diameter hysteroscopes. This has prompted the instrument manufacturers to develop sheaths which continue to have a final diameter of < 5 mm, but this now includes a working channel and continuous flow features (see Chapter 3). The new hysteroscopes enable diagnostic and operative hysteroscopy to be performed in the outpatient setting, without cervical dilatation and consequently without anaesthesia or analgesia. The advent of bipolar electrosurgical technology, for use with small-diameter hysteroscopes with working channels and continuous flow systems, has significantly changed the way we treat intrauterine pathologies and perform hysteroscopic procedures in a 'see-and-treat' fashion in the outpatient setting. The advantages of bipolar over monopolar technology in hysteroscopy are the use of saline solution rather than non-ionic distension media (*i.e.* glycine, sorbitol, mannitol, *etc.*), and the reduction of energy spread through the tissue during the procedure. Thus, new instruments using bipolar energy facilitate safe surgery (see Chapter 3).

This ambulatory, hysteroscopic, diagnostic and treatment service has been of great interest to healthcare universities, teaching hospitals and community-based diagnostic centres. For the first time anywhere in the world, nurses have been trained to carry out outpatient hysteroscopy in a pioneering course under the leadership of the authors who are recognised as pioneers of direct access outpatient hysteroscopy. This trend is likely to spread world-wide. See Table 2.1 for relevant definitions of concepts.

Table 2.1. Definitions

Outpatient services	Designed to serve as a resource for patients with conditions that do not require admission to hospital and overnight care
Ambulatory services	Ambulatory services are health services provided either in hospital outpatient clinics (*i.e.* patients who have NOT been admitted to hospital) or in primary care clinics
This book uses the above two terms interchangeably	
One-stop clinic	The traditional gynaecology clinic often involves several visits for consultations and investigations before the initiation of therapy. The one-stop clinic provides same-day investigations including haematology, pelvic ultrasound scan, hysteroscopy and endometrial biopsy. This allows prompt diagnosis and initiation of treatment
Rapid access	Accessible to general practitioners or other consultants from same or different specialties to avoid long waiting times, *e.g.* Postmenopausal Bleeding Clinic
Direct access	Readily accessible service to general practitioners or nurse practitioner in primary care without having to refer to a traditional outpatient clinic. Women are referred for just diagnosis and management, and then returned to primary care. The term is used interchangeably with rapid access, but is less commonly used
Fast track	Fast track referral system for patients with suspected gynaecological cancers who should be seen within a maximum of 2 weeks
This book uses the above four terms interchangeably	

Women with abnormal uterine bleeding should be assessed in a dedicated clinic offering pelvic scanning, hysteroscopy and tissue sampling at the initial visit. A gynaecologist usually staffs the one-stop clinic although, recently, nurse specialists have taken on the same role. Women are seen only once, though more time is needed to discuss findings and management options.

Outpatient techniques for hysteroscopy and suction sampling of the endometrium should be available in all units. Facilities to perform hysteroscopy and curettage under general anaesthetic are available for when the outpatient procedure is not possible or the patient has a strong preference for a general anaesthetic.

Recently published research has provided clinicians with high-quality data regarding the accuracy of ultrasonography and hysteroscopy in the diagnosis of endometrial disease. Despite this, controversy remains regarding the relative roles of these imaging and visualisation modalities. Services should consider including a component for audit and research, and should include provision for training juniors.

ADVANTAGES OF A ONE-STOP HYSTEROSCOPY CLINIC

An ideal one-stop clinic is an inclusive outpatient, ambulatory, rapid-access, see-and-treat clinic. It can be set up for a wide range of conditions. Common gynaecological conditions such as abnormal uterine bleeding are ideal for assessment in a one-stop clinic. Recent randomised trials have shown that this approach is efficient, and results in increased patient satisfaction.

The principal aim of investigations in the one-stop clinic is to identify or exclude endometrial pathology, most notably endometrial carcinoma. It is also important to ensure that women are sufficiently re-assured following normal tests, that symptomatic benign disease is identified, and that the process of investigation is both acceptable and efficient. Rapid alleviation of anxiety has been observed in women attending a one-stop clinic for assessing abnormal uterine bleeding problems.

Outpatient hysteroscopy offers many potential benefits over its traditional inpatient counterpart including faster recovery, less time away from work and home, cost savings to the woman and her employer and the health service. Resources need to be made available to develop these services and this book will serve as a guide to the various steps required for development of a One-stop Hysteroscopy Clinic.

Outpatient hysteroscopy brings significant benefits to the patient, the gynaecologist and the hospital as a whole.

Benefits to the patient

- There was a tendency toward improved diagnostic accuracy with ambulatory hysteroscopy for both endometrial cancer and disease compared to inpatient procedures
- Faster access to diagnosis and treatment
- Reduced delays and steps in the treatment process
- Faster return to normal functioning and work
- Improved patient satisfaction – there is constant communication with the gynaecologist throughout the procedure and the patient can follow the process visually if she wishes
- Safety – bipolar systems of electrosurgery are safer than monopolar systems. Thermal spread is minimised and distension of the uterus with normal saline reduces complications.

Benefits to the clinician

- More rapid identification of malignancy

- Excellent visualisation of the uterine cavity and clear operating field
- Opportunity to increase day-case rates
- Opportunity to protect elective activity from erosion due to rising medical emergency admissions
- Opportunity to run 'double' clinic sessions with a nurse practitioner.

Benefits to the hospital

- Reduction in cancer diagnosis waiting times
- Free-up capacity in wards and theatres for operation waiting list reductions and emergency work
- Potential to reduce diagnostic errors
- Increase day-case operation rates
- Hysteroscopy in a day-case or outpatient environment, using a see-and-treat model, lends itself to a direct-access, booked-admissions policy, streamlining patient flow
- Diagnostic hysteroscopies are also performed by Advanced Nurse Practitioners, Clinical Nurse Specialists or General Practitioners reducing the need for consultant input which can be used to better effect in more complicated operative hysteroscopic procedures.

HOW TO SET UP A ONE-STOP HYSTEROSCOPY SERVICE

The key merit of the one-stop service is to increase the activity through an outpatient setting, effectively enabling those patients who are found to have polyps, fibroids and small adhesions to have these treated at the same procedure. In order to introduce this into existing clinics, adjustments to the number of patients per session will be necessary, as operative procedures will take longer. This will

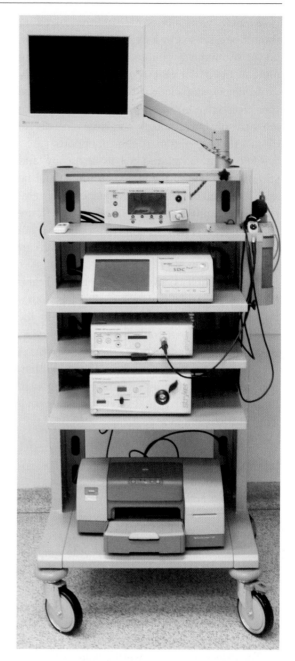

Figure 2.1. A mobile trolley with all the required units and video equipment.

increase the choices available to women, as they will get the option of 'see-and-treat' at diagnosis.

The room

Endoscopic procedures require a clearly arranged room setting. A well-organised room is crucial for the successful outcome of the procedure, for time saving and cost reduction. The service can be carried out in a normal outpatient consulting room if spacious enough to accommodate all necessary equipment and units. The room should be furnished and equipped to the standard of a minor surgery room (*e.g.* endoscopy) and should have a gynaecology operating chair. A mobile cart carrying all necessary units and video equipment (Fig. 2.1) can be used in the clinic.

A tray containing the instruments used for outpatient hysteroscopy should be set in a way that makes these instruments easily accessible. These instruments include: a sponge forceps, a volsellum, an os finder, a pack of 5 counted sterile surgical 4 x 5-inch gauze and a container for the disinfectant (Fig. 2.2). Before starting surgery, it is essential to check the instrumentation: the insufflation unit, light source, continuous-flow system: electrosurgical generator and the video camera system. Patients can recover in a normal waiting area or separate room.

Staffing

The operator (doctor or specialist nurse – Advanced Nurse Practitioner or Clinical Nurse Specialist) is assisted by one nurse who is in charge of the control of the instruments before and during the procedure (irrigation/suction system and electrosurgical generator). It is also essential to have an additional nurse or health care assistant whose role in supporting the patient is invaluable. Talking to the patient distracts her attention from the procedure.

All members of the clinical staff must be adequately trained and capable of solving all technical problems which might arise during the procedure.

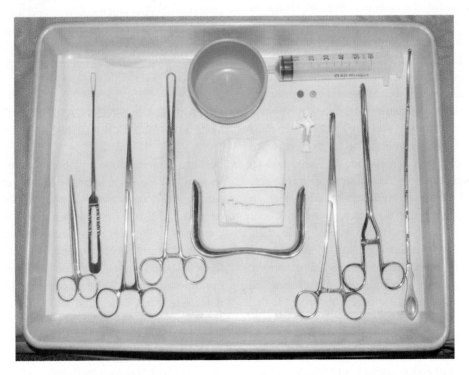

Figure 2.2. Tray containing the instruments used for outpatient hysteroscopy arranged to be easily accessible.

Positioning of patient

Figure 2.3 shows the positioning of patient, operator, nurse, health care assistant and the key pieces of equipment. It is of utmost importance to evaluate carefully the surgeon's interactive ability with the instruments in use. Thorough knowledge of the instrumentation and devices allows the surgeon to overcome any dysfunctions or malfunctions which are frequently encountered in hysteroscopy and may delay the intended examination or procedure.

Maintenance of hysteroscopy instruments

Dedicated facilities will be needed adjacent to the hysteroscopy room for washing, disinfection and sterilisation of instruments and endoscopes. Ideally, there should be separate sinks for washing and rinsing instruments. There should also be a separate hand basin for the operator. Staff in charge of cleaning, sterilisation, and maintenance of the instruments should be adequately trained and aware of the delicate nature and cost of the endoscopic instrumentation. Re-usable surgical instruments must be disassembled prior to cleaning. After decontamination, every (even small) part of the instrument and any hidden space must be cleaned with water and dried with compressed air. Alcohol or special soap should be used to clean lenses and telescopes. The operating instruments must be cleaned immediately after use in accordance with the manufacturer's instructions and these can be sent for steam sterilisation. Disposable instruments minimise the risk of transferring micro-organisms, including prions, between patients. Most modern instruments are designed for autoclave sterilisation at 134°C; however, some endoscopes involve fibre-optic technology and can not be autoclaved. The Medical Devices Agency (MDA) guidelines in the UK state that fibre-optic endoscopes are unable to withstand normal autoclave temperatures (121–137°C) and,

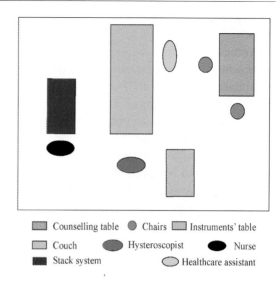

▭ Counselling table	● Chairs	▭ Instruments' table
▭ Couch	⬭ Hysteroscopist	● Nurse
▮ Stack system	⬭ Healthcare assistant	

Figure 2.3. Room set-up for outpatient hysteroscopy.

therefore, require immersion in disinfectants or sterilisation using gaseous processes such as ethylene oxide. The MDA suggests using 2% activated alkaline glutaraldehyde and lists suitable options including chlorine dioxide (i.e. Tristel).

A brief overview of sterilisation systems currently available is provided in Table 2.2.

PREPARING A BUSINESS CASE FOR A ONE-STOP HYSTEROSCOPY CLINIC

Business planning documentation may be required to justify a case for setting up a hysteroscopy service. The document should make a good impact on first sight. It should be persuasive and well presented giving facts and evidence for which this book will be an excellent source. Needless to say, the text should be free from spelling, grammatical or numerical errors. It should cover the key issues highlighted in Table 2.3, and the necessary supporting information. To ensure that local colleagues and managers support the proposal, the advantages of the business case for hysteroscopy should be unambiguous and supported by relevant and meaningful figures, wherever possible.

Table 2.2. Common sterilisation options

Chemical sterilisation

This is performed by immersing the instruments and endoscopes in a 2% glutaraldehyde solution. This solution may inactivate hepatitis B, hepatitis C, and human immunodefficiency viruses after a 20-minute immersion. However, to ensure complete sterilisation, a 10-hour immersion is required. This procedure is time-consuming and damaging to some instruments. If pre-operative screening is carried out to identify patients infected with hepatitis B, hepatitis C, and human immunodefficiency viruses, the respective patients could be excluded or scheduled in a special operative list. Then sterilisation by 20-minute immersion in a glutaraldehyde solution is a safe procedure

Autoclave sterilisation

This is the most inexpensive system. Unfortunately, instruments containing plastic parts, such as lenses and endoscopes, cannot be sterilised in autoclaves. For telescopes and instruments exclusively manufactured and sold as autoclavable, sterilisation cycles of 121°C for 20 minutes or 134°C for 7 minutes can be used

Gas sterilisation with ethylene oxide

This is an ideal system because it is carried out at low temperature and does not damage the endoscopic instruments. Unfortunately, this technique is expensive, time-consuming (72 hours before the instruments can be re-used), and requires the centre to have several sets of hysteroscopic instruments available. Therefore, only a few clinics use gas sterilisation

---

Table 2.3. List of headings for developing a business case for an ambulatory hysteroscopy service

Executive summary

Background
- The clinical problem – abnormal uterine bleeding and its diagnosis and treatment
- Patient demography – gathering relevant data and health-needs assessment on local patients is essential to evaluate the burden of disease due to abnormal uterine bleeding in the population that the primary healthcare team will serve
- Description of current services provided and the premises

Strategic context
- Drivers for change – clinical targets achievable and the obvious advantages of an ambulatory approach
- Objectives – to improve care for women with abnormal uterine bleeding
- Benefits expected from the change

Development proposal:
- Description of the options – ambulatory versus inpatient hysteroscopy

Preferred option
- Reasons for choosing the ambulatory option with a full option appraisal considering benefits to patients, staff and hospital with the cost of this option compared to inpatient hysteroscopy

Details of the proposed development
- Space requirements in square metres and site layout, capacity for future expansion, car parking requirements, etc. all need be considered

Continued on next page

Table 2.3. *(Continued from previous page)* List of headings for developing a business case for an ambulatory hysteroscopy service

Details of other partners in the proposed development
- Include histopathology and ultrasound departments citing evidence of track record and success of collaboration

Financial implications and affordability
- Discuss the costs compared to the benefits/value for money, estimated total project capital cost of the scheme and how the cost has been estimated. Achieve balance between income and expenditure with input from hospital management

Funding options
- There are several sources of funding but emphasise that you are looking at ways of doing things differently, not ways of using extra resources. Emphasise the potential savings from reducing multiple visits by the patients to hospitals, less complaints, less paperwork, *etc.*

Non-financial impact
- The main reason for the change is an improvement in quality. Try to quantify the likely impact of the change on key performance targets, *e.g.* waiting times that the organisation is judged by

Timetable

Management arrangements

Risk assessment
- An assessment of any factors that are likely to have a significant impact on the scheme, health and safety issues, *etc.* Why the proposed change will work? Also include potential risks and how to prevent them.

Conclusions, key benefits and outcomes
- Summarise the main beneficial aspects of the development of ambulatory hysteroscopy service: quality of care, staff morale, operational aspects such as faster response to enquiries to patients, communications, *etc.*

Appendices
- Include details which are best provided separately rather than within the main body of the bid document, *e.g.* financial calculations, *etc.*

Key points

➢ Ambulatory (outpatient) hysteroscopy does not require an overnight hospital stay.

➢ The aim of the investigations of abnormal uterine bleeding is to diagnose endometrial cancer, hyperplasia and benign pathology.

➢ Ambulatory hysteroscopy in a one-stop clinic is efficient and results in increased patient satisfaction due to the rapid alleviation of anxiety, faster recovery, and less time away from work and home.

➢ The key merit of the one-stop clinic is to increase the throughput in an outpatient setting effectively giving women the option of treatment at diagnosis, *i.e.* 'see-and-treat'.

➢ Ambulatory hysteroscopic procedures require a clearly arranged room setting, staffing (medical and nursing members) and lead clinician.

➢ For establishing a one-stop hysteroscopy service, a business case may have to be prepared.

3 Equipment required for ambulatory hysteroscopy

OBJECTIVE: To provide a detailed overview of the equipment and instruments needed to perform a hysteroscopy in the ambulatory setting, both diagnostic and operative.

CONTENTS

INTRODUCTION

In 1869, Pantaleoni performed the first outpatient hysteroscopy, diagnosing an endometrial polyp and cauterising it with silver nitrate. A second generation of endoscopes was developed by Nitze in 1879 who constructed a cystoscope with a lens system and a light source inside the endoscopic tube. With this innovation, vision was clearer, lighting was more intense and the field of vision was wider.

Improvements in distension media took place in the early 1970s. Performing hysteroscopy using CO_2 resolved some of the difficulties that prevented the wide-spread use of hysteroscopy. The new, improved visual optics and fine-diameter instruments (4 mm) achieved in the 1980s and 1990s revolutionised the field of hysteroscopy. Technical innovations in hysteroscopic equipment have led to easy performance of comprehensive examination, and simple treatments in the ambulatory setting without anaesthesia or cervical dilatation.

STACK SYSTEM AND ROOM SET-UP
(see also Chapter 2)

Outpatient hysteroscopy is usually performed in a room with limited space. A mobile stack system (see Fig. 2.1) carrying all the equipment is, therefore, required and is positioned so that the surgeon has a good view of the monitor and the equipment displays (see Fig. 2.3). Knowledge of the room set-up, available instruments, and assisting staff are crucial for successful ambulatory hysteroscopy. Music and relaxing images might play a part in relieving patients' anxiety.

The set-up of the room should always be checked prior to starting the clinic. This includes testing the camera, light source, distension media and other mechanical and bipolar instruments. A named nurse should be in charge, at all times, of cleaning, sterilising and maintaining the instruments according to unit policy. This person should be adequately trained and fully aware of the delicate nature and the cost of the hysteroscopic equipment.

HYSTEROSCOPES

A panoramic hysteroscopic view should be obtained by using either a rigid or flexible hysteroscope. While rigid endoscopes have two versions (the single flow and the continuous flow systems), flexible scopes are only available as single flow instruments.

Flexible hysteroscopes

The flexible hysteroscope was developed to overcome difficulties in viewing the cornual areas and in entering an acutely anteverted and retroverted uterus. It is a safe, successful, and reliable method of investigating abnormal uterine bleeding in the ambulatory setting. The flexible hysteroscope is composed of three main parts:

1.   The proximal end that contains the ocular system, distal manipulator, opening to the operating channel, exit site for the operating sheath and light source.

2.   Flexible sheath, which contains the fibre-optic bundles and the operating channel.

3.   The distal end, which can bend to 100° on both sides of the longitudinal axis.

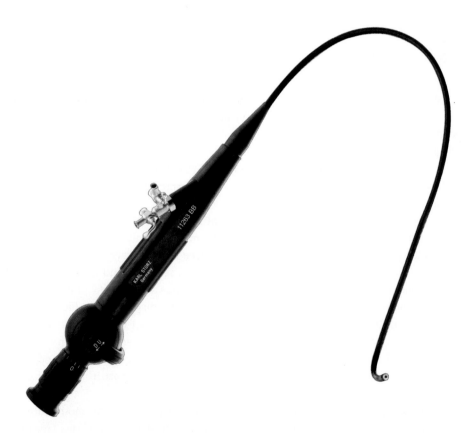

Figure 3.1 A typical flexible hysteroscope.

When compared with rigid hysteroscopy, flexible hysteroscopy is believed to be associated with less pain both at introduction of the hysteroscope and during the procedure itself especially when using a smaller diameter scope. However, flexible systems have not become wide-spread because of their high cost, fragility and difficulty in sterilisation (Fig. 3.1).

Rigid hysteroscopes

Three types of rigid lens systems are in common use – Hopkins, Lumina and Olympus. Technical improvements aim at maintaining high resolution at various distances and with various magnifications. Rigid telescopes are available in different angles of vision ranging from 0° (180°) to 30° (150°, forward-oblique), the former being the most popular for office hysteroscopy. Their external diameters vary from 1.2 mm to 4 mm. Telescopes are focused at infinity; therefore, magnification is inversely proportional to the distance of the object from the lens. As the 30° telescope passes through the cervical canal with axis aimed at the symphysis pubis, the internal cervical os appears lower in the field of view than where it actually lies (Fig. 3.2).

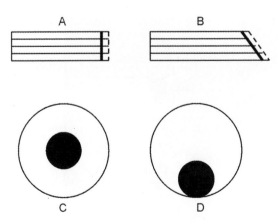

Figure 3.2. Diagrammatic representation of 0° and 30° telescopes (A,B) and the view of cervical canal during the introduction of the hysteroscope (C,D).

The telescope is inserted into an examination sheath, which can be a single inflow sheath with one stopcock or a continuous flow sheath. An outer sheath of < 5 mm diameter is considered preferable for outpatient use as it allows examination without anaesthesia or cervical dilatation (Fig. 3.3a–c).

Single flow system

These scopes are commonly used in the outpatient setting. The diameter of the diagnostic outer sheath is < 4 mm. The flow of CO_2 or saline, which is introduced into the space between a single flow sheath and the telescope, creates the desired distension of the uterine cavity.

Double (continuous) flow system

Distension with a continuous flow of liquid requires a double sheath for infusion and aspiration. For optimal fitting in the internal cervical os, the sheath should preferably have a round circumference. Continuous liquid flow is indicated in patients with bleeding because it can maintain a clear vision.

LIGHT SYSTEM

High-quality light is an indispensable component of outpatient hysteroscopy, as it should be performed under video-endoscopic vision.

Light source

Satisfactory sources of 'cold' light using halogen or xenon are available. Xenon light is the most commonly used due to its characteristic illumination, which is close to sunlight. The power required varies from 100 W to 300 W. In general, 175 W is sufficient to obtain a satisfactory view. Higher power is used for special inter-

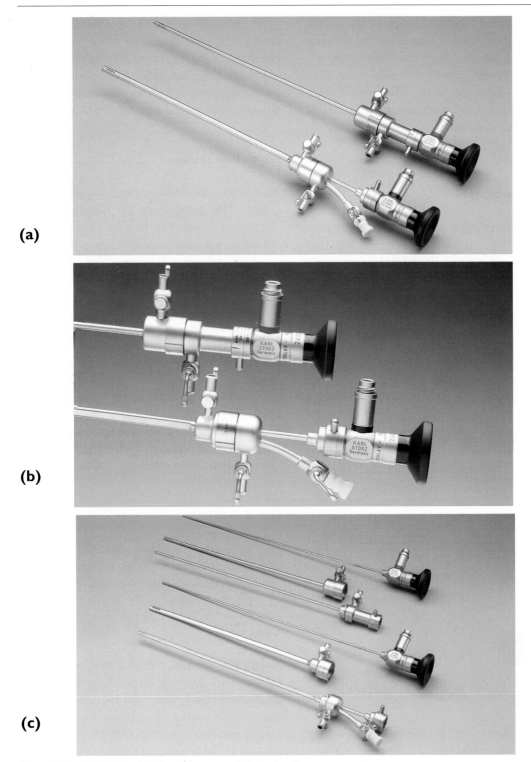

(a)

(b)

(c)

Figure 3.3(a–c). Various rigid hysteroscopes and their sheaths.

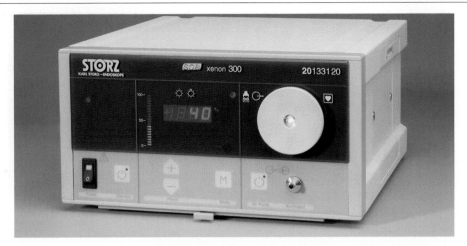

Figure 3.4. Power source for a xenon light source.

vention or filming. With increasing light power, there is an associated heat production and an increase in the temperature (Fig. 3.4).

Light cable

A fibre-optic light cable consists of densely packed longitudinal bundles of glass fibres, with diameter between 3.5–4.5 mm and length between 180–350 cm that transmits light from the source to the telescope (Fig. 3.5).

CAMERA

In the outpatient setting, a video camera should always be in use as it facilitates examination in a comfortable position (Fig. 3.6a,b). The head of the camera is attached to the eyepiece of the telescope and a video image is displayed on the colour monitor. A video camera consists of a lens and either one or three solid-state integrated circuit image sensors referred to as CCDs (charge coupled devices) or chips. In a single-chip camera, one-third of the pixels (photosensitive cells) are

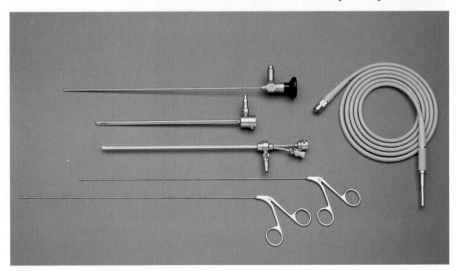

Figure 3.5. Rigid hysteroscope with associated fibre-optic light cable.

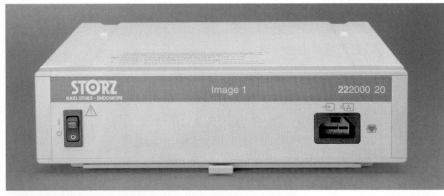

(a)

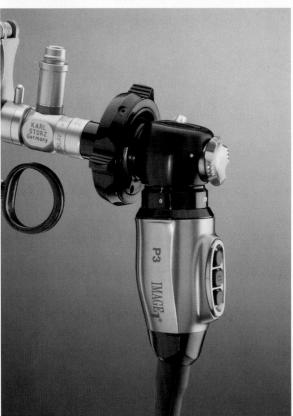

(b)

Figure 3.6(a,b). Hysteroscope with camera fitted and its associated electronic unit.

devoted to each colour (red, green or blue). The camera then generates the colour electronically. However, in the three-chip cameras, each chip is devoted to a single colour and each chip detects the entire image. Three-chip cameras have an increased colour separation, high resolution and decreased picture noise. However, they are expensive in comparison with the single-chip versions.

A good camera combines the characteristics of high resolution, good quality of video output/images and a high signal-to-noise ratio. The later ensures that image quality will remain constant with changing conditions such as bleeding. With advancing technology, cameras are now available in small, light-weight versions with focusing ring, zoom feature and automatic adjustments for gain, brightness and white balance.

DISTENSION MEDIA

Adequate uterine cavity distension is a fundamental prerequisite to obtaining a panoramic view. Distension media differ according to whether the hysteroscopic procedure is diagnostic or operative. Several methods are in use including carbon dioxide (CO_2) gas and low viscosity fluids (dextrose, lactated Ringer's buffer, glycine, sorbitol, or saline solution).

Carbon dioxide (CO_2) distension medium

Carbon dioxide is a colourless gas that is rapidly absorbed and cleared easily from the body by respiration. It can be used safely for outpatient hysteroscopic purposes. A steady flow of CO_2 allows even uterine cavity distension. In order to keep a safe and constant flow of CO_2, a pre-set hysteroflator, which automatically maintains pressure at 100–120 mmHg with a flow of 30–60 ml/min should be used. The controlled flow of this gas keeps the intra-uterine pressure between 40–80 mmHg.

With large quantities or uncontrolled delivery of CO_2, gas embolism can result in serious complications. However, the levels of CO_2 used during an entire hysteroscopic examination are far less than those that produce significant toxicity. Disadvantages include: (i) creation of air bubbles, which could obscure the view especially if there is bleeding; (ii) shoulder tip pain in some women due to gaseous irritation of the diaphragm; and (iii) CO_2 is unable to clear the uterine cavity of debris in comparison with fluid media.

Low-viscosity distension media

Low-viscosity fluids such as dextrose (5–10%), dextran (4–6%) and saline solutions can also be used to produce uterine distension for diagnostic purposes. However, as these solutions are electrolyte based, they are considered unsuitable for procedures that require the use of monopolar electric current. In contrast, saline is ideal for bipolar electrosurgery.

Different techniques are adopted to create sufficient pressure for adequate uterine distension. A fluid bag positioned at 90–100 cm above the patient's couch creates a pressure of 65–75 mmHg. A pressure cuff positioned around the bag and inflated to 80 mmHg is commonly used in outpatient hysteroscopy. The use of an electronic pump for infusion/aspiration allows the creation of a continuous flow in the uterine cavity that maintains a constant, clear view with proper uterine distension. The HAMOU Endomat is an example of the latter pump system and is usually set-up at 70 mmHg outflow pressure and 0.25 bar suction pressure. Nowadays, normal saline is commonly used for uterine distension in office hysteroscopy. It is easily available at low cost. A randomised study comparing CO_2 with saline, as distension media for outpatient hysteroscopy, concluded that both media are comparable in terms of overall patient discomfort levels and satisfaction but saline provides superior views.

HYSTEROSCOPIC ACCESSORIES

Semi-rigid mechanical, re-usable instruments (*e.g.* scissors, snares, grasping and biopsy forceps) are available for outpatient use (Fig. 3.7).

VERSASCOPE AND VERSAPOINT

The Versascope is a semi-rigid hysteroscope for use in outpatient settings. A small diameter hysteroscope (1.8 mm), with a working length of 28 cm and a 0° lens, allows a field of view of 75° (Fig. 3.8a). A disposable outer sheath (continuous flow system) of 3.5 mm contains an expandable working channel for instruments up to 2 mm diameter (5 French). The channel also accomodates a bipolar electrode. The system is supplied with a digital camera system that rotates 360° for full peripheral view while maintaining proper orientation. Xenon light (175 W) is used to provide illumination. A compact ceramic xenon lamp enables the light source to achieve high output and uniform illumination without hot spots (Fig. 3.8b). Energy is delivered from the generator to the tissue through the active electrode. This causes immediate cellular rupture and vaporisation. The energy then passes through the saline to the return electrode and back to the Versapoint generator (Fig. 3.8c). It can cut, coagulate, vaporise and desiccate small intra-uterine lesions such as polyps, focal adhesions, small pedunculated submucous myoma, and small uterine septa. The system operates by a contact technique that enables continuous visualisation of tissue effect. This allows instan-taneous tissue vaporisation without the need to eliminate resection chips.

This innovation is very useful in ambulatory and office operative hysteroscopy because the electrodes fit easily into the 5-F (1.6 mm) operating

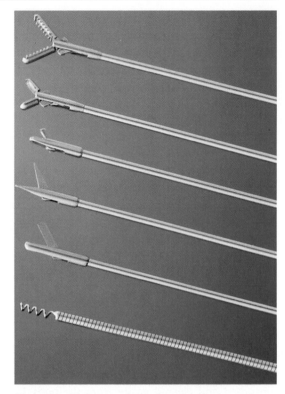

Figure 3.7. Various mechanical accessories for use in hysteroscopy.

channel available on most hysteroscopes used for outpatient hysteroscopy. Another advantage is that it can be used with physiological saline as a distension medium thus reducing the chance of fluid overload when compared with use of

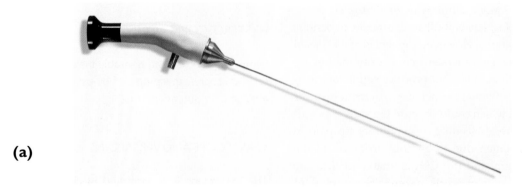

(a)

Figure 3.8. (*See next page for details*)

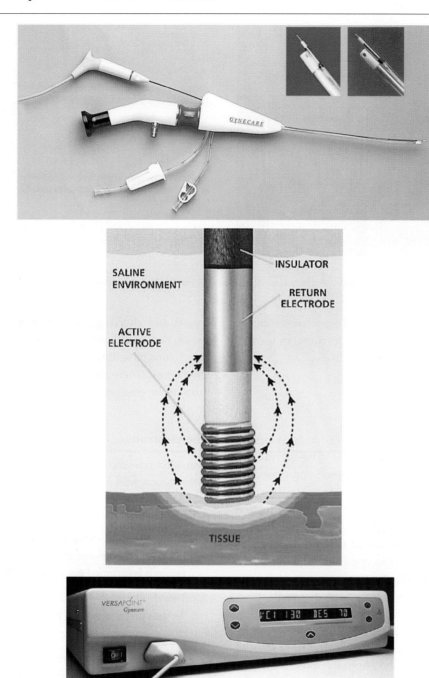

Figure 3.8. (a) The Versascope; (b) with accessories; and (c) the dedicated generator for bipolar electrosurgery. Note: (i) consolidation of active and return electrodes into single instrument; (ii) current is symmetrically distributed throughout the tissue between the electrodes; (iii) patient is not part of the essential current pathway; (iv) thermal damage is limited to a discrete volume of tissue; and (v) power requirements are reduced with higher electrosurgical efficiency.

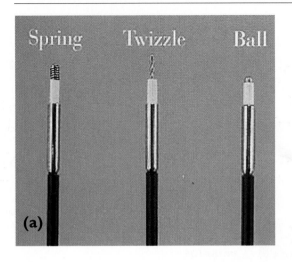 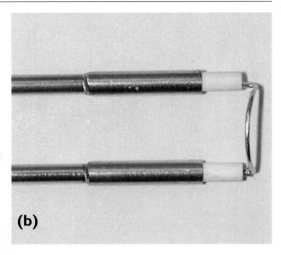

Figure 3.9. (**a**) Spring, twizzle and ball electrodes: (**b**) the Versapoint bipolar loop electrode.

hypotonic non-ionic media like glycine, sorbitol or mannitol when monopolar electrosurgery is used. Lateral thermal spread is less likely.

The technology

Energy is delivered via a generator to tissues through the active electrode. The active and return electrodes are 'staggered' or placed in line with a ceramic insulator or spacer between them. Both a modulated and non-modulated current can be employed giving the bipolar electrode the versatility to cut and desiccate as in monopolar electrosurgery with the safety of a bipolar coagulating forceps.

As the electrode is activated, small steam bubbles form into a 'vapour pocket' which, upon contact with the tissue, causes instantaneous cellular rupture. When the tissue comes into contact with the vapour pocket, the tissue forms part of a return circuit. Tissue adjacent to the vapour pocket has increased resistance. The current seeks the path of least resistance – through the saline distension medium to the return electrode and back to the energy generator (Fig. 3.8c); hence, minimal lateral thermal

spread and charring. The generator has three, preset, non-modulated current settings and two blend current settings and one modulated current setting. There are several in-built safety features in the generator.

The electrodes

Four electrode configurations are available. Any hysteroscope with a 5–7 Fr (1.6–2.0 mm) operating channel will take any of the three bipolar electrodes described below (Fig. 3.9a)

1. **Spring electrode** – has a large surface suitable for tissue vaporisation and debulking. Fibroid vaporisation is best carried out using this electrode.

2. **Twizzle electrode** – for cutting tissues. Suitable for resecting endometrial polyps, treating intracavitary fibroids, dividing septa and adhesions.

3. **Ball electrode** – allows precise tissue vaporisation and desiccation. Suited for haemostasis (rarely used in clinical practice).

4. **Versapoint bipolar loop electrode** (Fig. 3.9b) – for use under general anaesthetic to resect endometrial polyps, fibroids or endometrium (used with a standard resectoscope).

Key points

➤ Knowledge of the room set-up, available instruments, and assisting staff is crucial for successful outpatient hysteroscopy.

➤ Flexible hysteroscopy is believed to be associated with less pain both at introduction of the hysteroscope and during the procedure.

➤ Rigid hysteroscopes are available with viewing angles of 0–30°. Their external diameters vary from 1.2 mm to 4 mm and are in more frequent use.

➤ Three-chip cameras are better than single chip ones because of improved picture quality.

➤ CO_2 and saline are comparable in terms of overall patient discomfort and satisfaction but saline provides superior views.

MULTIPLE CHOICE QUESTIONS

1. **The flexible hysteroscope**

   Helps to overcome difficulties in viewing the cornual areas   True/False

   Helps in entering acutely anteverted and retroverted uterus   True/False

   Cannot be used in ambulatory setting   True/False

   When compared with rigid hysteroscopy, it is believed to be associated
   with more pain   True/False

2. **Rigid hysteroscopes**

   Are available in different angles of vision ranging from 0° to 30°   True/False

   Their external diameters vary from 5 mm to 7 mm   True/False

   Magnification is inversely proportional to the distance of the
   object from the lens   True/False

   Continuous liquid flow is indicated in patients with bleeding   True/False

3. **Distension media**

   Carbon dioxide is a gas that is rapidly absorbed and cleared easily from the
   body by respiration   True/False

   CO_2 can be used only in the inpatient setting   True/False

   Shoulder tip pain is one of the postoperative disadvantages   True/False

   Air bubbles could obscure the view   True/False

4. **Low viscosity distension media**

Dextrose (5–10%), dextran (4–6%) and saline solutions all are low-viscosity
distension media   True/False

They are considered suitable for the use of monopolar electric current   True/False

Normal saline is commonly used in office hysteroscopy   True/False

Comparing CO_2 and saline, both media are comparable in terms of overall
patient discomfort, satisfaction and clarity of view   True/False

5. **The Versascope**

Is a small diameter hysteroscope (1.8 mm) in a disposable outer
sheath of 3.5 mm   True/False

Contains a working channel for instruments up to 2 mm in diameter   True/False

Uses a monopolar electrode   True/False

Is very useful in ambulatory and office operative hysteroscopy   True/False

4 Basic hysteroscopic technique

OBJECTIVE: To provide an overview of a basic diagnostic hysteroscopic technique in the outpatient setting.

CONTENTS
Procedures for diagnostic hysteroscopy
Endometrial sampling
Failed hysteroscopy

Role of transvaginal sonography
Key points
MCQs

PROCEDURES FOR DIAGNOSTIC HYSTEROSCOPY

Hysteroscopy has long been considered as merely a visual method of investigation; today, thanks to recent advances in instrumentation, diagnostic techniques have been modified to allow simultaneous use of the telescope and surgical instruments. Miniaturised instruments have enabled the clinician not only to perform targeted hysteroscopic biopsies, but also to treat benign intra-uterine pathologies, such as polyps and synechiae, without any premeditation or anaesthesia. This has been defined as a 'see-and-treat' procedure: there is often no distinction between the diagnostic and operative procedures, but a single procedure in which the operative part is perfectly integrated in the diagnostic work-up.

Consent

Before performing hysteroscopy, seeking a patient's consent, verbal or written, is an ethical obligation. Successful relationships between clinicians and patients come from respecting patients' autonomy, effective communication and building trust. In obtaining consent, one has to ensure that the patient is given adequate information for consent and all questions are answered. Clinicians should give a clear explanation of the scope of consent being sought. This book does not recommend the patient's apparent compliance as a form of consent. For example, the fact that a patient lies down on an examination couch does not, in itself, indicate that the patient has understood what hysteroscopy is and why it might be needed. Clinicians must fully discuss all the information required for women to make an informed decision in language that is easily understood and, if necessary, translations should be provided.

The consent should be obtained by the clinician who will perform the hysteroscopy. Clinicians should give clear explanations about: (i) what is the procedure; (ii) the purpose of the procedure; (iii) the likelihood of positive and

Table 4.1. Patient information leaflet/frequently asked questions

What is hysteroscopy?

Hysteroscopy provides a way to look inside the womb or uterus and is an outpatient procedure. A hysteroscope is a thin, telescope-like instrument with light transmission. It is inserted through the vagina and cervix (neck of the womb). Sometimes, the procedure is simply for diagnostic purposes allowing determination of whether there are any abnormalities such as fibroid, polyps, scar tissue, a uterine septum, or some other uterine problem. At other times, the procedure is used for treatment purposes, such as the removal of a tissue sample, polyp or fibroid. The hysteroscope is generally 2.5–5.5 mm in diameter. The actual procedure takes 2–5 minutes and no anaesthesia is needed for most cases of diagnostic hysteroscopy. If hysteroscopic treatment is required, then local anaesthesia may be used.

How long does it take?

With this procedure, the patient is discharged home about 15–30 minutes after completion.

When can I return to work?

Return to work or resuming normal daily activities by the next morning (if local anaesthesia was used) or immediately (if no anaesthesia or local was used) is the norm. Mild pain and cramping is common after treatment hysteroscopy, but is usually brief (lasting perhaps 30 minutes, occasionally up to 8 hours).

What are the reasons for performing hysteroscopy?

The reason for hysteroscopy depends on the type of problem. Some frequent indications for hysteroscopy are:

- Hysteroscopy may be used to confirm the results of other tests such as ultrasonography and hysterosalpingography such as a polyp or a septum
- Women of child-bearing age with period problems unresponsive to medical treatment
- Women of child-bearing age with break-through bleeding on hormone replacement therapy (HRT)
- Women of child-bearing age with infertility or recurrent abortions
- Women of child-bearing age with a misplaced intra-uterine contraceptive device
- Women with postmenopausal bleeding
- Suspected endometrial cancer
- Breast cancer patients who are receiving Tamoxifen and who develop uterine bleeding

When should hysteroscopy be performed?

The best time for hysteroscopy is during the first week or so after your period. During this time, your physician is best able to view the inside of the uterus.

How hysteroscopy is performed?

Patient lies down and is positioned well down on the operating table to ensure the buttocks overhang the end of the table. The gynaecologist sits between the patient's legs. The patient is draped; her vulva and introitus area are thoroughly cleaned. A speculum is inserted to locate the cervix. The gynaecologist may then gently dilate the cervix. After adequate dilatation, a hysteroscope is inserted slowly through cervix. For good vision, a balanced flow of saline is started to clean and wash out blood and tissue debris. Once the hysteroscope enters the uterine cavity, either saline or CO_2 is used to distend the uterus. When the hysteroscope gives a good view of the interior of the uterus, gross pathology can be detected. After complete examination, the hysteroscope is gently withdrawn and the vagina is cleaned.

(continued on next page)

Table 4.1.*(continued)* Patient information leaflet/frequently asked questions

What are the complications of hysteroscopy

Most patients will probably have nothing more than a mild lower abdominal pain after the procedure. Possible complications of hysteroscopy include bleeding and puncture of the uterus (uterine perforation). Bowel damage may occur after uterine perforation. However, such complications are rare. If it happens, a diagnostic laparoscopy (key-hole surgery) should be performed to examine any possible bowel injury. If there is no bowel injury and the uterine perforation is small (as is usually the case), then the patient can be discharged the next day with antibiotic coverage. In case of a large perforation and extensive bowel injury, open operation may be necessary but this is extremely rare.

negative findings, including false-negative and false-positive results; (iv) uncertainties and the possibility of not reaching a diagnosis due to poor views and risks of the procedure; and (v) follow-up plans (if there will be any). This will allow patients sufficient time to reflect before and after they make a decision. Leaflets (Table 4.1), given to patients and general practitioners about the procedure beforehand, can enhance and underpin the consent. They help in decision making by allowing extra time at home to discuss with other family members. Clinicians should be prepared to discuss fully with the patient all the issues in Table 4.2; basically, what the procedure is likely to involve, and the benefits and risks of any available alternative treatments, including no treatment. The

Table 4.2 Consenting for hysteroscopy

1. **Describe the nature of hysteroscopy and explain the procedure** as described in the patient information leaflet, *i.e.* it is a vaginal approach involving insertion of a hysteroscope through the cervix.

2   **Any additional proposed procedure** (such as endometrial biopsy, removal of a polyp, insertion of a levonorgestrel-releasing intra-uterine system, treatment of fibroids or division of adhesions) must be discussed and consent obtained

3   **Serious or frequently occurring risks**. It is recommended that clinicians make every effort to separate serious from frequently occurring risks. Women who have had previous uterine surgery (lower segment caesarean section, myomectomy) or cervical surgery (cone biopsy) should understand that risks will be increased

   Serious risks include
   Uterine perforation (8 per 1000)
   Pelvic infection
   Failure to visualise uterine cavity

   Frequent risks include
   Vaginal bleeding and discharge
   Pain: either pelvic or shoulder

   Any extra procedures which may become necessary during the examination
   Laparoscopy in the event of perforation
   Blood transfusion (very rare)

Table 4.3. When making video recordings

1. Seek permission to make the recording and get consent for any use.

2. Give patients adequate information about the purpose of the recording.

3. Ensure that patients are under no pressure to give their permission for the recording to be made and that withholding permission will not affect the quality of care they receive.

4. Stop the recording if the patient asks.

5. Ensure that the recording does not compromise patients' privacy and dignity. Do not use recordings for purposes outside the scope of the original consent for use, without obtaining further consent.

6. Make appropriate secure arrangements for storage of recordings.

7. Obtain permission to make and consent to use any recording made for reasons other than the patient's treatment or assessment (recordings made for the training or assessment of doctors, audit, research or medicolegal reasons).

8. After the recording, patients should be given the chance, if they wish, to see the recording, and to vary or withdraw their consent to the use of the recording. They should understand that recordings are given the same level of protection as medical records against improper disclosure.

role of endometrial biopsy and pelvic ultrasound should be discussed along with the option of no investigation. A record should be made of the information leaflet/tape given to the woman prior to surgery.

When making recordings of hysteroscopy, clinicians must take particular care to respect patients' autonomy and privacy. Table 4.3 shows the general principles that apply to most recordings.

Clinical assessment

History taking (age, parity, menopausal status, use of hormone replacement therapy, cervical smear history and past history of cervical or uterine surgery) and examination (general, abdominal and vaginal) are essential steps in the clinical assessment of patients before hysteroscopy. Conducting pelvic examination allows an assessment of the uterus, its position (anteverted, retroverted), its mobility and also the adnexae.

Patient positioning

Care when positioning of the patient is important to prevent musculoskeletal and neurological complications. Hysteroscopy is performed in the lithotomy position with legs apart supported in leg rests with the buttocks a few centimetres extending beyond the end of the table. The back should be flat on the table, not flexed, to avoid postoperative lower-back discomfort. No joint in the leg should be flexed over 60° to avoid femoral nerve compression (associated with extreme flexion, abduction, and lateral rotation at the hip). Avoiding excessive pressure on the lateral aspect of the lower legs within the stirrups helps avoid perineal nerve compression.

Adjustment of speculum and positioning of hysteroscopist

Consideration of the findings of the physical examination will help in directing the speculum

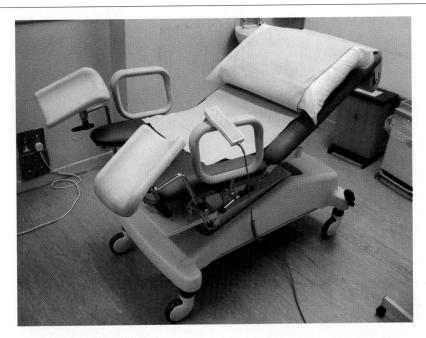

Figure 4.1. The hysteroscopy couch.

to enable the hysteroscopist to visualise the cervix with ease. The speculum should be directed posteriorly if the uterus is anteverted or anteriorly if the uterus is retroverted. In acutely anteverted uterus, the patient's bed should be positioned higher; in acutely retroverted uterus, it should be lower (Fig. 4.1). This allows easier instrumentation by the hysteroscopist, whose chair should be easily adjustable too.

Vaginal disinfection and analgesia

A sterile speculum is inserted to visualise the cervix which is gently cleansed with antiseptic. Outpatient hysteroscopy is a relatively painless procedure that may take only a few minutes. Diagnostic, outpatient hysteroscopy is performed without anaesthesia; for operative hysteroscopy, local anaesthetic is injected into the cervix and premedication with analgesia is required (usually a non-steroidal anti-inflammatory, e.g. diclofenac).

This combination usually provides adequate relief of the discomfort/cramping pains that can be experienced during dilating the cervix and uterine distension in an operative hysteroscopic procedure. If local anaesthetic is to be used, the cervix may be injected with local anaesthetic or a local anaesthetic gel (Instillagel) may be instilled into the canal. The preparation, the dose, and the site of injection are discussed in detail in Chapter 5. However, most cases should need neither local anaesthetic nor tenaculum or forceps to grasp the cervix for diagnostic procedures.

Vaginoscopy

Outpatient hysteroscopy with a semi-rigid 2.5-mm hysteroscope using the vaginal speculum and cervical tenaculum is a well-tolerated and successful technique for the evaluation of abnormal genital tract bleeding, but any attempt to minimize pain in the ambulatory setting is welcomed by patients.

Vaginoscopy is an approach (without speculum or tenaculum) that may eliminate patient discomfort related to the traditional approach to examine the vagina and cervix. With the patient in the lithotomy position, the hysteroscope is introduced into the vagina. Using the hysteroscope, the vagina is distended using normal saline solution at a pressure of 50 mmHg. There is no need to close the interoitus. The vagina is inspected with the hysteroscope and the vaginal walls can be visualised thoroughly. The hysteroscope is then introduced into the posterior vaginal fornix and then gently withdrawn until the cervix come into view. The hysteroscope is then introduced into the cervical canal and the pressure is decreased to 25 mmHg. Vaginoscopy procedure is now complete and the hysteroscope is gently guided into the uterine cavity to carry on with the standard hysteroscopy procedure.

Vaginoscopy is easy to perform and incurs no additional cost. It is ideal for office hysteroscopy and in patients who otherwise might require general anesthesia just because they cannot tolerate a vaginal speculum, such as virgins and older women with somewhat stenotic vaginas. Continuous-flow vaginoscopy using the hysteroscope and normal saline for irrigation and distension is very quick, easy and efficacious.

Hysteroscopy

As a general principle, the hysteroscope should always be the first instrument to be inserted into the cervical canal. Dilatation of the cervical canal and probing of the cavity are not necessary. If bleeding occurs in the canal as a result of sounding, it may interfere with hysteroscopic inspection of the uterine cavity. Exceptions to this are in cases of cervical stenosis due to ageing, cervical surgery, or conisation. In these situations, one can use the os finder to negotiate the cervix or a thinner diameter hysteroscope. Local application of prostaglandins may be used to soften the cervix (Table 4.4).

The tip of the hysteroscope (30°, 0°, rigid or flexible; see Chapter 3) is gently placed in the external cervical canal. The distension medium is turned on, allowing time for hydrodilatation where the fluid dilates before the scope (the distension medium will be turned off before removal of the scope from the canal). The hysteroscope is then introduced into the cervical canal and advanced under direct vision into the uterine cavity. Normal saline solution or carbon dioxide gas are used to distend the endometrial cavity to improve visualisation and to flush away any bleeding or debris. A light source is

---

Table 4.4 Prostaglandin to prime the cervix

- The efficacy of misoprostol for cervical ripening before first-trimester suction curettage abortion is well established.

- Vaginal misoprostol in doses of 200, 400 or 800 µg, may be used 4 hours before a hysteroscopic operative procedure.

- Some studies have used sublingual misoprostol 100 µg, 12 hours' pre-operatively.

- The available evidence suggests that vaginal misoprostol lessens the cervical resistance in women undergoing hysteroscopy and facilitates the procedure; however, benefit is not certain.

- This evidence is mainly for hysteroscopy in premenopausal women. Further research to demonstrate the benefit of using misoprostol as a cervical ripening agent in postmenopausal women is needed.

- Reported side effects include nausea, vomiting, diarrhoea, dizziness, headache, fever, chills, rashes, and pelvic pain.

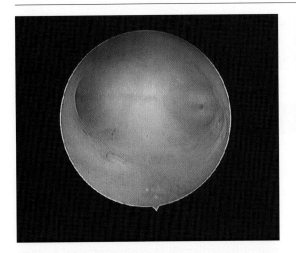

Figure 4.2. Normal uterine cavity.

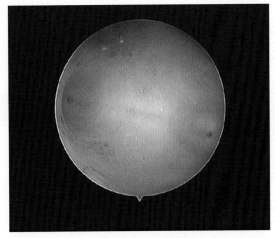

Figure 4.3. Both ostia seen.

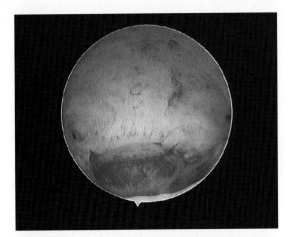

Figure 4.4. Both ostia seen with endometrial polyp.

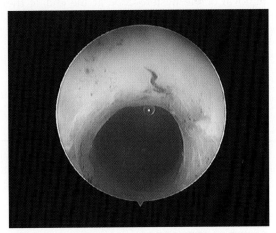

Figure 4.5. Normal cervical canal.

also attached to the scope to illuminate the uterine cavity. A camera system should be used for training purposes and for patient involvement.

During examination of the ectocervix, low magnification provides an excellent view of the cervix, a step that should never be missed. However, traditional colposcopy presents clear advantages because the colposcope allows a more accurate observation of fine vascular details. Low-magnification hysteroscopy gives a panoramic view and can provide important information on the integrity of the anatomical structure of the cervical canal. During the examination of the uterine cavity, simple panoramic viewing at x20 magnification has proved extremely useful in identifying the shape of the uterine cavity, any irregularities and all types of endometrial pathology. The ostia of the Fallopian tubes and endometrium can be inspected. Endometrial tissue samples may be removed for pathological examination (Figs 4.2–4.5).

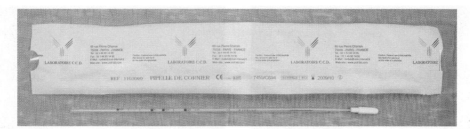

Figure 4.6. Pipelle endometrial sampler.

Once the hysteroscope has been inserted through the cervical canal, the fundus, the tubal ostia (the main points of orientation in the uterine cavity), and the walls of the cavity may be assessed in a stepwise fashion. Assessment of the cervical canal may be carried out best on the removal of the hysteroscope at the end of the diagnostic procedure.

ENDOMETRIAL SAMPLING

Histological specimens may be obtained either at the same time as hysteroscopy (directed/target) or using a blind endometrial suction sampling device, e.g. Pipelle (Fig. 4.6). Research has demonstrated that such sampling has a high degree of accuracy for diagnosis of endometrial cancer and hyperplasia.

FAILED HYSTEROSCOPY

Hysteroscopic procedures unable to make a final diagnosis because of technical aspects (*e.g.* cervical stenosis, anatomical factors, structural abnormalities), inadequate visualisation (*e.g.* obscured by bleeding, debris) or patient factors (*e.g.* pain, intolerance) are categorised as failed procedures. Problems such as pain, bleeding, poor endoscopic vision, or poor distension of the uterine cavity are directly related to the experience of the hysteroscopist and patient tolerance.

The failure rate for an ambulatory procedure varies between 2–8% in the literature (around 4%)

which is no different from that of an inpatient procedure. In failed procedures, endometrial disease may be present in around 3% of cases. The failure rate of hysteroscopy in postmenopausal women is no higher than in premenopausal women. Potentially serious complications like pelvic infection, uterine perforations, bladder perforation, and cardiovascular episodes occur in 2–3 per 10,000 hysteroscopy patients (see Chapter 8 for details). The inadequate specimen rate on endometrial biopsy is around 5%.

ROLE OF TRANSVAGINAL SONOGRAPHY

Patients referred to the one-stop outpatient hysteroscopy clinic with abnormal uterine bleeding may also have a transvaginal ultrasound scan. In postmenopausal women, the mean endometrial thickness is much thinner than in premenopausal women. Thickening of the endometrium (≥ 4 mm) may indicate the presence of pathology. In general, the thicker the endometrium, the higher the likelihood of important pathology (endometrial cancer) being present. Transvaginal ultrasonography can reliably assess thickness and morphology of the endometrium and can thus identify a group of women who have a thin endometrium and are, therefore, unlikely to have significant endometrial disease. This group may not require any further investigation unless there is a recurrence of bleeding. The relatively non-invasive nature of transvaginal ultrasonography may make it more acceptable

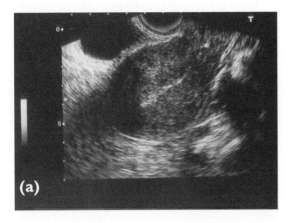 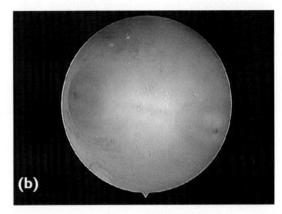

Figure 4.7. (a) Thin endometrium on transvaginal sonography; (b) atrophic endometrium on hysteroscopy.

than other investigations. Those patients with thickened endometrium require further investigations in the form of hysteroscopy and endometrial sampling. Figure 4.7a,b shows thin endometrium on transvaginal sonography corresponding to atrophic endometrium on hysteroscopy. Figure 4.8a,b illustrates thick endometrium on transvaginal sonography corresponding to endometrial hyperplasia on hysteroscopy.

In premenopausal women with abnormal uterine bleeding, there are numerous reasons for symptoms. The endometrium undergoes cyclic changes in response to ovarian steroid hormone stimulation. During these changes, the thickness of the endometrium varies, and it becomes difficult to establish guidelines as to what should be considered 'normal' thickness. Thus, it can be difficult to establish a diagnosis particularly if women do not have regular cycles. Saline-enhanced transvaginal ultrasonography for endometrial texture and margin analysis can be used to help improve diagnostic accuracy. Other ultrasonographic techniques such as transvaginal Doppler ultrasonography, and three-dimensional

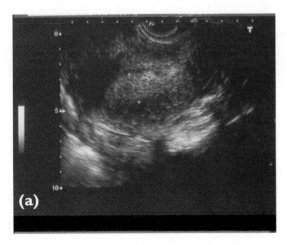 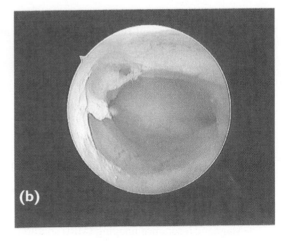

Figure 4.8. (a) Thick endometrium on transvaginal sonography; (b) endometrial simple hyperplasia on hysteroscopy.

ultrasonography are also being gradually introduced for improving discrimination between anomalies (*e.g.* polyps versus fibroids). There is no evidence to support their introduction into routine clinical practice at present.

In summary, ambulatory hysteroscopy is safe with a low incidence of serious complications. It has a small failure rate which is unaffected by menopausal status.

There is a general consensus that hysteroscopy is the current gold standard in studying and evaluating intra-uterine anatomy and pathology, including submucous myomas, polyps, hyperplasia and cancer. Hysteroscopy in the outpatient setting appears to have an accuracy and patient acceptability equivalent to inpatient hysteroscopy under general anaesthetic.

Key points

➢ Diagnostic outpatient hysteroscopy is usually performed without any anaesthesia or analgesia.

➢ The hysteroscope should always be the first instrument to be inserted into the cervical canal. Dilatation of cervix is not necessary in a majority of cases.

➢ For hysteroscopy, the tubal ostia are the main points of orientation in the uterine cavity.

➢ A panoramic view of the endometrial cavity allows an assessment of abnormalities.

➢ Assessment of the cervical canal on removal of the hysteroscope captures cervical pathology.

➢ Ambulatory hysteroscopy is safe, accurate in diagnosis and acceptable to patients.

MULTIPLE CHOICE QUESTIONS

1. **In postmenopausal bleeding, what is the most likely diagnosis?**

Atrophic vaginitis	True/False
Endometrial polyp	True/False
Endometrial hyperplasia and carcinoma	True/False
Cervical polyp and cancer	True/False
Adnexal malignancy	True/False

2. **In the initial investigation of women with postmenopausal bleeding:**

Transvaginal ultrasound scan has a high sensitivity	True/False
Outpatient hysteroscopy is the investigation of choice	True/False
Magnetic resonance imaging (MRI) should be used if available	True/False
Pelvic examination can be replaced by transvaginal ultrasound scan	True/False

3. **In postmenopausal bleeding:**

Outpatient endometrial biopsy is often necessary — True/False

A pelvic ultrasound scan is performed for endometrial thickness measurement and adnexal masses — True/False

Outpatient hysteroscopy allows direct visualisation of the uterine cavity — True/False

Inpatient dilatation and curettage is required routinely — True/False

4. **In obtaining the consent for hysteroscopic procedure:**

The consent should be obtained by any member of the team — True/False

Clinicians do not breach confidentiality when they disclose information with their patients' consent — True/False

Patients should give separate consent for information about them to be shared among healthcare professionals — True/False

The valid consent of a competent patient can only be given by the patient — True/False

5. **When making video recordings of hysteroscopy:**

Clinicians may not take consent for it — True/False

Withholding permission will not affect the quality of care patients receive — True/False

Using recordings for purposes outside the scope of the original consent needs further consent — True/False

Patients should understand that recordings are given the same level of protection as medical records against improper disclosure — True/False

5 Pain control in outpatient hysteroscopy

OBJECTIVE: To provide a detailed analysis of pain management in relation to outpatient hysteroscopy.

CONTENTS

Anatomical considerations
Why hysteroscopy causes pain and discomfort
Anaesthetic techniques for outpatient hysteroscopic procedures

Analgesia for hysteroscopy
Key points
MCQs

Outpatient hysteroscopy is being increasingly used as a first-line investigation for abnormal uterine bleeding and other conditions involving the uterine cavity. The main limitation to its wide-spread use in the past has been low patient tolerance due to pain. Providing anaesthesia and analgesia is a clinical challenge. The goal of ambulatory hysteroscopy is to provide an effective investigation with a comfortable experience for the patient.

ANATOMICAL CONSIDERATIONS

The innervations of the uterine body and uterine cervix is best understood by reviewing the anatomical features of the neural network in the pelvis (Fig. 5.1). The presacral space begins at the bifurcation of the aorta into the iliac arteries. Lying on the sacrum, with the middle sacral vessels, is the pelvic autonomic nervous system, the presacral nerve plexus (or the superior hypogastric plexus). It divides into two nerves, the right

and left hypogastric nerves, that lead to the inferior hypogastric nerve plexus. This collection of nerves lies just lateral to the uterus and vagina in the uterosacral/cardinal ligament complex. This plexus contains sympathetic pelvic splanchnic nerves from the thoracolumbar trunk and para-sympathetics from the craniosacral trunk. It has three portions: (i) the vesical anterior plexus; (ii) the uterovaginal plexus (also known as Frankenhauser's or Lee-Frankenhauser's plexus); and (iii) the middle rectal plexus.

It is the Frankenhauser's plexus that appears to innervate the lower part of the uterine body, the cervix, and the upper vagina. It lies on the dorso-medial surface of the uterine vessels, just lateral to the uterosacral/cardinal ligament complex. The uterine vessels, within the cardinal ligaments, enter the cervix at the 3- and 9-o'clock positions. An additional set of nerves may also be contained within the uterosacral complex that insert at the 4- and 8-o'clock position on the posterior aspect of the uterus. It has been debated whether all of the innervations of

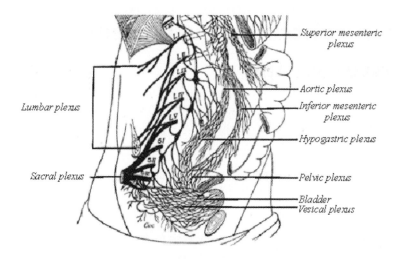

Figure 5.1. Innervation of the uterus. [Figure details from Fig. 838 in Henry Gray. *Anatomy of the Human Body*, 1918. Reproduced from www.bartleby.com with the permission of Bartleby]

the uterine body are truly from Frankenhauser's plexus. Other possibilities include collateral neural connections from the infundibulopelvic ligament, which contains the ovarian neurovascular bundle. This may be particularly true as it relates to the uterine body.

WHY HYSTEROSCOPY CAUSES PAIN AND DISCOMFORT

The International Association for the Study of Pain gives this definition: 'pain is an unpleasant sensory and emotional experience associated with actual or potential tissue damage'. Distension of the uterine cavity causes discomfort and pain. The lower the distension pressure in the uterus, the less the discomfort: a minimum of 30 mmHg is needed to separate the uterine walls. In the outpatient setting, the pressure should be kept to this minimum and increased only if the view is poor. A prospective, randomised clinical trial comparing carbon dioxide and normal saline for uterine distension in outpatient hysteroscopy found significantly less abdominal pain and less shoulder tip pain with

saline. Irrespective of the distension medium used, pelvic discomfort is worse in nulliparous women than in multiparous women. The size of hysteroscope and sheath has an impact on pain and success rates. Diameters of less than 3.5 mm are well tolerated in the outpatient setting. Addition of endometrial biopsy to hysteroscopy increases pain.

The menopause has no effect on the procedure being painful. Talking to the patients during the procedure distracts them and allows the patient to focus on another subject; hence, the role of a well-trained nurse (Auxiliary, Healthcare Assistant) in attendance.

ANAESTHETIC TECHNIQUES FOR OUTPATIENT HYSTEROSCOPIC PROCEDURES

It is important to remember that the majority of outpatient diagnostic hysteroscopy cases do not need any anaesthesia or analgesia. One can remove polyps or treat fibroids with minimal pain when using bipolar energy snares or mechanical instruments. It is only required if there is a need to

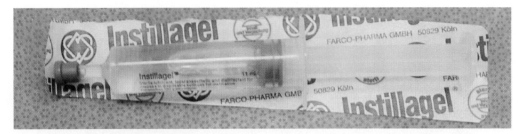

Figure 5.2. Instillagel (CliniMed) Gel, lidocaine hydrochloride (2%).

overcome cervical stenosis, *i.e.* to dilate the cervix, or during outpatient operative hysteroscopy.

Providing anaesthesia, in cases where standard procedures outlined in Chapter 4 are uncomfortable, is a clinical challenge. The available techniques for outpatient endometrial procedures include topical lignocaine spray or Instillagel, intra-uterine lidocaine, the traditional paracervical block, the deep paracervical block, and conscious sedation. Each offers some benefit in providing pain relief during these procedures.

Topical anaesthesia to cervix

The value of local anaesthetic agents applied to the ectocervix is in pain reduction with tenaculum application, but this technique does very little to provide anaesthesia for the endometrial portion of the procedure. Typically, the anaesthetic is applied via a spray. For example, 10% lignocaine spray may be administered to the ectocervix, and then a tenaculum may be applied. The nozzle of the spray canister can then be threaded into the cervical canal so that the endocervical canal and potentially the endometrial cavity would be exposed. An example is the Xylocainex (AstraZeneca) Spray (a pump spray) containing lidocaine (10%; 100 mg/ml) supplying 10 mg lidocaine/dose with 500 spray doses per container. A total of 10 metered doses were given to each patient in one study which indicated a limited value of this therapy. Limited absorption into the endometrial cavity may explain the failure of this technique to control pain.

Intracervical lidocaine injection in outpatient hysteroscopy can also reduce cervical sensitivity, but it is insufficient to block uterine stimuli resulting from distension and manipulation of the uterine cavity. Topical application or intracervical injection of lignocaine is beneficial only for tenaculum placement. It is important not to forget that most diagnostic hysteroscopy procedures do not require application of a tenaculum to the cervix.

Intra-uterine instillation of anaesthesia

Intra-uterine administration is proposed to deliver anaesthesia to the uterine cavity. Medication is injected using a flexible catheter placed deeply into the endocervical canal or directly into the endometrial cavity (Fig. 5.2). Lidocaine is allowed to sit in the cavity; through absorption, anaesthesia is achieved. This technique was found not to disrupt the histological architecture of the endometrial specimen in one study. Randomised trials have shown that, with pain scales, there is a statistically significant reduction in pain with the use of intra-uterine lidocaine compared to saline. One must wait at least 3–5 minutes before performing hysteroscopy after instillation of anaesthetic in the uterine cavity for it to give effect.

Doses of anaesthetics for intra-uterine instillation

Lidocaine (Lignocaine 2%; 20 mg/ml; use 5 ml) is effectively absorbed from mucous membranes and is a useful surface anaesthetic in con-

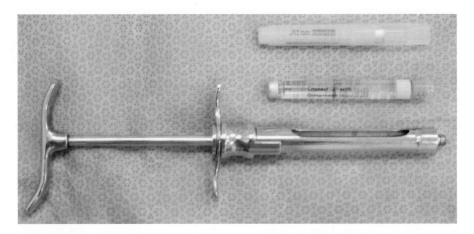

Figure 5.3. Prilocaine hydrochloride (Citanest®): injection 1%(10 mg/ml). Prilocaine is a local anaesthetic of low toxicity which is similar to lidocaine (lignocaine). Doses to a maximum of 400 mg may be used. If used in high doses, methaemoglobinaemia may occur which can be treated with intravenous injection of methylthioninium chloride (methylene blue) 1% using a dose of 1 mg/kg.

centrations of 2–4%, except for surface anaesthesia; solutions should not usually exceed 1% in strength.

Use of vasoconstrictors

Most local anaesthetics, with the exception of cocaine, cause dilatation of blood vessels. The addition of a vasoconstrictor such as adrenaline (epinephrine) diminishes local blood flow, slows the rate of absorption of the local anaesthetic, and prolongs its local effect. Adrenaline must be used in a low concentration (1 in 200,000; 5 μg/ml) for this purpose. The total dose of adrenaline should not exceed 500 μg and it is essential not to exceed a concentration of 1 in 200,000 (5 μg/ml) if more than 50 ml of the mixture is to be injected.

Paracervical block

The traditional paracervical block involves injection of 1–2 ml of local anaesthetic solution (prilocaine, Citanest®) superficially into the tenaculum site at 12-o'clock (Fig. 5.3). Then the cervix is gently grasped. Injections of 1–2 ml are used superficially to create blebs around the cervico-vaginal mucosa with a total of 10 ml to create a ring around the cervix. Further 10-ml boluses are injected deeply into the lower uterine segment where the uterosacral ligaments attach (4-quadrant block). By pulling the cervix forward, one can see 'tenting' at the ligament attachment. The paracervical block involves injecting deeply using the full length of the 1.5-inch needle at 2- and 3-o'clock and between 4- and 5-o'clock on the one side and then at 9- and 10-o'clock and between 7- and 8-o'clock on the other. Aspiration before injection is essential. One soon learns the amount of resistance present when the needle is correctly placed. If the needle is outside the uterus, there is no resistance; if the needle is too close to the internal os, there is more resistance than in the myometrium of the lower uterine segment.

The technique, widely used by inexperienced clinicians for endometrial outpatient procedures, often does not involve deep paracervical block. Instead, the injecting anaesthetic is just placed at the cervico-vaginal reflection. Research studies including randomised trials among women undergoing hysteroscopy and endometrial biopsy have shown that only with using the deep injection technique does a statistically significant improvement in pain management become apparent. It is unclear whether the afferent pain fibres from the uterine body run in Frankenhauser's plexus or whether they are included in the neurovascular bundle of the infundibulopelvic ligament. The technique of deeply embedding the needle in the lower uterine segment at the paracervical nerve plexus is effective and safe as it is without serious complications. Based on these observations, only the paracervical block using the deep injection technique is a beneficial tool to reduce pain in hysteroscopic procedures.

Conscious sedation with intravenous medications

Conscious sedation is defined as an arousable, but drowsy, state in which a patient is able to maintain verbal contact and an airway. This is differentiated from general anaesthesia and deep sedation, which are depressed states of consciousness or unconsciousness accompanied by partial or complete loss of protective reflexes. Using conscious sedation converts the case into a day-case procedure, not an ambulatory or outpatient procedure, because the patient needs monitoring during hysteroscopy and a subsequent recovery phase. Details of this method fall beyond the scope of this book. A randomised study comparing local anaesthesia with conscious sedation for outpatient bipolar operative hysteroscopy has concluded that conscious sedation is without significant differences in terms of pain control and patient satisfaction.

ANALGESIA FOR HYSTEROSCOPY

Analgesia, in the form of paracetamol or a non-steroidal anti-inflammatory drugs (*e.g.* diclofenac) may be used for ambulatory hysteroscopic operations. One-hour before the procedure, women may be given 100 mg of diclofenac-sodium suppository. In recent years, the non-steroidal anti-inflammatories have been extensively used for outpatient hysteroscopic procedures and, in most studies, have demonstrated high efficacy. They are particularly useful at these ambulatory settings because of their simplicity of administration and low incidence of side-effects; they have, therefore, become particularly popular. They act by inhibiting the enzyme cyclo-oxygenase. Simple analgesics such as paracetamol orally 0.5–1 g every 4–6 hours to a maximum of 4 g daily may be added for analgesia following the procedure.

Key points

➢ Providing pain relief for outpatient hysteroscopic procedures remains a challenge in only a small proportion of patients. The majority of outpatient diagnostic hysteroscopy cases do not need anaesthesia. Usually, anaesthesia/analgesia is only necessary during outpatient operative hysteroscopy or if there is a need to dilate the cervix.

➢ The application of topical anaesthetic agents appears to have little or no added benefit for endometrial procedures, but can make the application of a tenaculum more comfortable for the patient.

➢ The deep injection technique for paracervical block provides most consistent pain relief.

(continued on next page)

Key points *(continued)*

➢ Analgesia, in the form of paracetamol and/or an non-steroidal anti-inflammatory, may effectively be used for ambulatory hysteroscopic procedures.

➢ Vaginoscopy is an approach that may eliminate patient discomfort related to the traditional approach. One of the key steps in vaginoscopy is passing the endoscope through the internal cervical os without speculum or volsellum (see Chapter 4).

MULTIPLE CHOICE QUESTIONS

1. **Regarding the innervations of the uterine body and uterine cervix:**

    The presacral space begins at the bifurcation of the aorta into the iliac arteries   True/False

    Lying on the coccyx, with the middle sacral vessels, is the pelvic autonomic
    nervous system   True/False

    The inferior hypogastric nerve plexus is a collection of nerves lying just lateral to
    the ovaries in the infundibulopelvic ligaments   True/False

    This plexus contains sympathetic pelvic splanchnic nerves from the
    thoracolumbar trunk and parasympathetics from the craniosacral trunk   True/False

2. **Regarding Frankenhauser's plexus:**

    It innervates the lower part of the uterine body, the cervix, and the upper vagina   True/False

    It lies on the dorso-medial surface of the uterine vessels, just lateral to the
    uterosacral/cardinal ligament complex   True/False

    The uterine vessels, within the cardinal ligaments, enter the cervix at the 3- and
    9-o'clock positions   True/False

    All of the innervation of the uterine body is truly from Frankenhauser's plexus   True/False

3. **Regarding pain and discomfort during hysteroscopy:**

    Distension of the uterine cavity causes discomfort and pain   True/False

    The higher the distension pressure in the uterus the more the discomfort   True/False

    A minimum of 60 mmHg is needed to separate the uterine walls   True/False

    The size of hysteroscope and sheath has no impact on pain and success rates   True/False

4. **Additional contributing factors to the pain:**

    Addition of endometrial biopsy to hysteroscopy increases pain   True/False

    Menopause has an impact on the procedure being painful   True/False

Talking to the patient is a recognised factor in distracting the women's attention during the procedure — True/False

Irrespective of the distension medium used, pelvic discomfort is worse in nulliparous women than in multiparous women — True/False

5. Regarding pain control in outpatient hysteroscopy:

The application of topical anaesthetic agents has a significant benefit — True/False

The deep paracervical block is of unproven efficacy — True/False

Analgesia, in the form of paracetamol and/or diclofenac may effectively be used for ambulatory hysteroscopic procedures — True/False

Vaginoscopy means passing the hysteroscope through the internal cervical os without speculum or volsellum — True/False

6. Ambulatory hysteroscopy

Is associated with severe pain in less than 10% of women — True/False

Has a failure rate of 8% of all attempted procedures — True/False

Anaesthesia is only required if there is a need to dilate the cervix — True/False

When using bipolar energy to remove polyps or treat fibroids, anaesthesia is essential — True/False

6 Indications and contra-indications for ambulatory diagnostic hysteroscopy

OBJECTIVE: To give an overview of indications and contra-indications for ambulatory diagnostic hysteroscopy.

CONTENTS

Indications for ambulatory diagnostic hysteroscopy	Key points
Contra-indications to ambulatory hysteroscopy	MCQs

INDICATIONS FOR AMBULATORY DIAGNOSTIC HYSTEROSCOPY

The benefits of carrying out a procedure must outweigh the potential risks and there must always be specific indications. The indications for outpatient hysteroscopy are many, as summarised in Table 6.1.

Abnormal uterine bleeding

Abnormal uterine bleeding is the commonest reason for hysteroscopic examination. Hysteroscopy is particularly useful in the investigation of the structural causes of abnormal uterine bleeding, as there is direct visualisation of the endometrial cavity. It allows direct, targeted biopsies of abnormal or suspicious looking areas of the endometrium and other lesions within the uterine cavity. Its usefulness is further enhanced when combined with other investigative techniques such as transvaginal pelvic ultrasonography and endometrial sampling.

Abnormal uterine bleeding can be sub-divided into: (i) premenopausal bleeding problems;

(ii) postmenopausal bleeding; and (iii) unscheduled bleeding on hormone replacement therapy or tamoxifen. Abnormal uterine bleeding accounts for more than 20% of referrals to the gynaecologist and accounts for 25% of gynaecological procedures in premenstrual women.

Prior to considering hysteroscopy, it is important to rule out pregnancy and pregnancy-related bleeding conditions in all women of child-bearing age. Other causes of abnormal uterine bleeding that need exclusion are anovulatory bleeding from conditions like polycystic ovarian disease, hyperprolactinaemia and thyroid disease, impending premature ovarian failure, bleeding from use of hormonal preparations (oral contraception, contraceptive implants and injections), bleeding diathesis (*e.g.* von Willebrand's disease), bleeding from infective causes (*e.g.* cervicitis, endometritis) and bleeding from complications of the use of intra-uterine contraceptive devices.

During the perimenopausal period, ovarian function diminishes and anovulatory bleeding is more likely to occur. However, one must be aware that, at this age, neoplastic pathologies such as endometrial hyperplasia and carcinoma

Table 6.1. Indications for outpatient hysteroscopy (diagnostic and operative)

- Evaluation of abnormal uterine bleeding

- Diagnosis and treatment of focal intra-uterine lesions, e.g. polyps, fibroids

- Investigation of infertility

- Diagnosis and treatment of intra-uterine adhesions

- Diagnosis and treatment of uterine septa

- Investigation of recurrent miscarriage

- Location and retrieval of lost intra-uterine contraceptive device (IUD) and foreign bodies

- Ablation of the endometrium

- Hysteroscopic sterilisation

are more common. Endometrial carcinoma is rare before the age of 40 years and its incidence rises steeply between ages 45–55 years. Between 5–10% of all women with postmenopausal bleeding will have endometrial cancer.

Structural lesions responsible for abnormal uterine bleeding are often at their peak during the perimenopausal period; these include focal lesions (*i.e.* endometrial polyps and submucous fibroids) and diffuse lesions (*i.e.* endometrial atrophy, hyperplasia, cancer and diffuse adenomyosis).

Endometrial hyperplasia and cancer

Endometrial hyperplasia is deemed a precursor of endometrial cancer. Diagnosis and classification of endometrial hyperplasia must be considered one of the primary goals of any early detection programme. The depth of mucosa can be evaluated by simple pressure with the end of the hysteroscope. In comparison with the normal, smooth, thin endometrium without vascularisation, features of increased endometrial thickness, abnormal vascularisation, and polypoid formations are considered the hysteroscopic features of hyperplasia (severe glandular with or without atypia). Mamillations

and cerebroid irregularities associated with irregular polylobular, friable excrescences with necrosis or bleeding are considered diagnostic hysteroscopic features of malignancy (Fig. 6.1a–c).

Other structural causes

These are infections (endometritis, pyometrium, tuberculosis, pelvic inflammatory disease), foreign objects (intra-uterine contraceptive devices), atrophic endometrium, Asherman's syndrome with partial occlusion of the outflow tract, Mullerian abnormalities and vascular (arteriovenous) malformations.

In the past during investigation of abnormal uterine bleeding, several diagnostic techniques have been used. Blind dilatation and curettage, endometrial biopsy using Vabra or Pipelle suction, hysterosalpingography, transvaginal ultrasound scan, *etc.* Blind dilatation and curettage only samples 60% of the endometrium; most focal lesions (polyps and fibroids), which will be obvious at hysteroscopy, are missed by dilatation and curettage. A large meta-analysis revealed that in both postmenopausal and premenopausal women, the Pipelle was the best device with cancer deletion rates of 99.6% and 91% respectively. Transvaginal

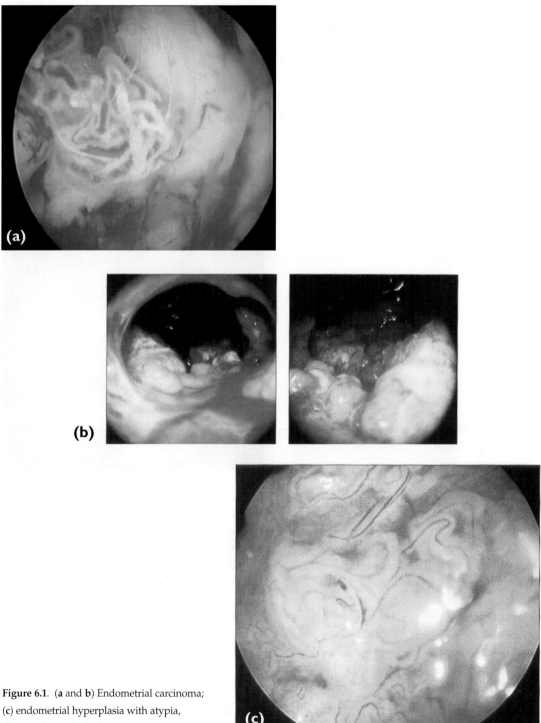

Figure 6.1. (**a** and **b**) Endometrial carcinoma; (**c**) endometrial hyperplasia with atypia, abnormal vascularisation.

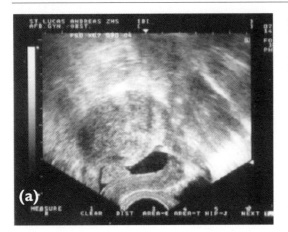

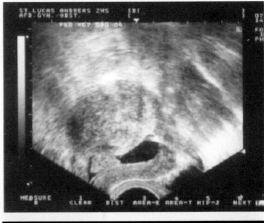

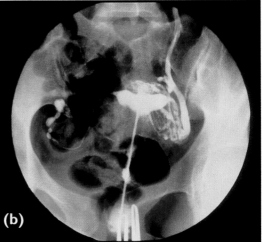

Figure 6.2. (**a**) Saline infusion sonography showing focal lesion [*with the permission of Andreas Thurkow*]; (**b**) hysterosalpingography.

measurement of endometrial thickness (a reproducible measurement) is better at predicting the risk of endometrial cancer in postmenopausal than perimenopausal women.

In a large meta-analysis of approximately 6000 women, the prevalence of endometrial cancer was 13% and the prevalence of endometrial polyps and hyperplasia was 40%. For women with postmenopausal bleeding, the best balance of sensitivity versus specificity is obtained at an endometrial thickness measurement of 5 mm – 92% and 81%, respectively.

Hysterosalpingography identifies some intracavitary lesions but is limited by its inability to identify diffuse lesions consistently. More recently, sonohysterography (saline infusion sonography) has been used to differentiate focal from diffuse endometrial lesions (Fig. 6.2a).

Outpatient hysteroscopy will diagnose all focal lesions (endometrial polyps and submucous fibroids), will aid targeted biopsy of suspicious and abnormal areas of the endometrium. When combined with pelvic transvaginal ultrasound and endometrial biopsy, it is invaluable in the investigation of abnormal uterine bleeding (*see* Chapter 4, Figs 4.7a,b and 4.8a,b).

Infertility

Hysteroscopy is not used routinely in the investigation of infertility. It is more common to

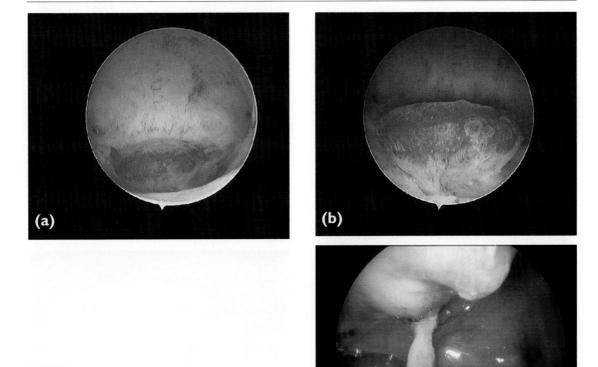

Figure 6.3. (**a** and **b**) Endometrial polyp; (**c**) pedunculated endometrial polyp.

use hysterosalpingography (Fig. 6.2b). Hysterosalpingography has a high false-positive rate due to transient distortion of the uterine cavity from mucus, debris, bubbles and blood. Hysterosalpingography has an 85–100% sensitivity in detecting tubal pathology in infertile patients but only 44% sensitivity in documented intra-uterine malformations and 75% in intra-uterine adhesions (synechiae).

The main indication for use of hysteroscopy in the investigation of infertility is in clarifying intra-uterine status when an abnormal hysterosalpingography result is obtained.

Outpatient hysteroscopy is the diagnostic procedure of choice in confirming and planning treatment for intra-uterine anomalies in infertile patients. It also permits the inspection of the cervical canal and the tubal ostia. Lesions detected by outpatient hysteroscopy in infertility investigations include endometrial polyps, submucous fibroids, intra-uterine adhesions (synechiae), and uterine septa.

Endometrial polyps

Ten percent of women presenting with infertility have endometrial polyps. There has been some suggestion that women with polyps have a higher rate of spontaneous miscarriage but there is no evidence of lower pregnancy rates in this group. Outpatient hysteroscopy easily identifies women with sub-fertility and endometrial polyps but the value of routine hysteroscopic removal of these polyps before fertility treatment is unknown (Fig. 6.3a–c).

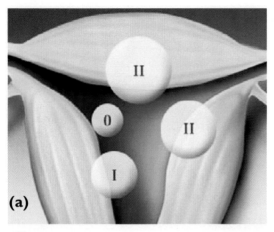

(a)

Type   Intramural extension
  0   None
  I   <50%
  II   >50%

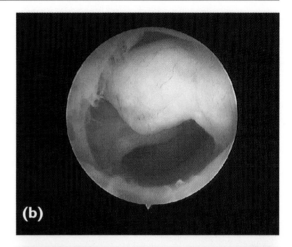

(b)

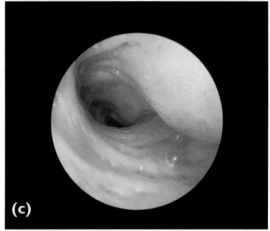

(c)

Figure 6.4.

(**a**) Submucous fibroids classification;

(**b**) submucous fibroid type I;

(**c**) submucous fibroid type II.

Fibroids

Fibroids have rarely been shown to be a direct cause of infertility. There is evidence to show that fibroids indirectly affect fertility because they alter the contractility of the uterus and may disrupt normal sperm migration. Fibroids may also affect the vascular and molecular profiles of sites of implantation and, in some cases, cause partial obstruction of the tubal ostia. Some studies indicate high success rates in both pregnancy and live births following removal of fibroids in women with otherwise unexplained infertility.

Submucous fibroids, type 0 and type I (Fig. 6.4a), distorting the uterine cavity are well placed for hysteroscopic diagnosis and removal (Fig. 6.4b–d). Most authors recommend removal of fibroids no more than 2 cm in diameter in the outpatient setting. The commonest instrument in use is the bipolar spring electrode.

Intra-uterine synechiae (Asherman's syndrome)

This is usually a result of intra-operative or postoperative complications occurring during uterine evacuation, termination of pregnancy or hysteroscopic surgery. It can also be caused by uterine infections like schistosomiasis and mycobacterium. Asherman's syndrome has been found in 13% of women undergoing routine infertility investigations. Typical symptoms are menstrual

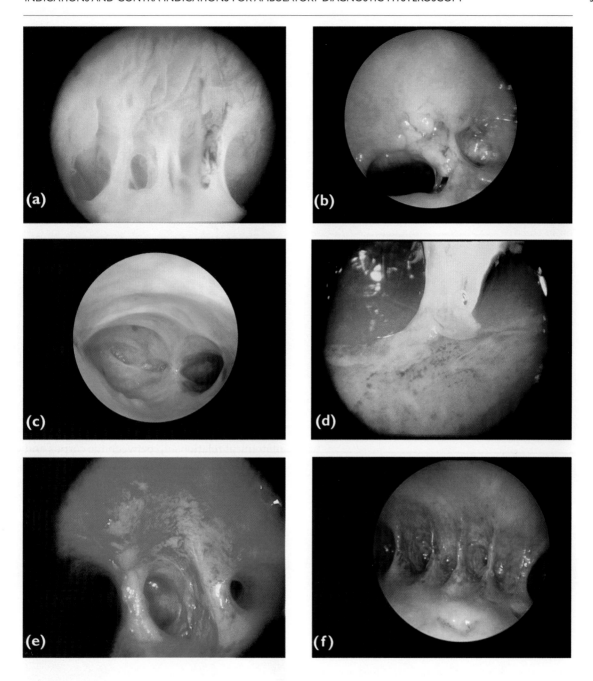

Figure 6.5. (a–f) Intra-uterine synechiae (Asherman's syndrome).

irregularities, amenorrhea, and miscarriage.

Outpatient hysteroscopy is ideal for the detection of intra-uterine adhesions (Fig. 6.5a–f).

Treatment can be offered using mechanical instruments or a bipolar 'twizzle' electrode in the outpatient setting.

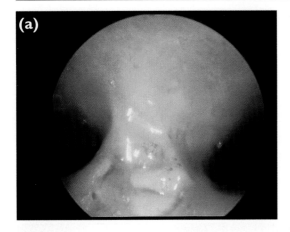

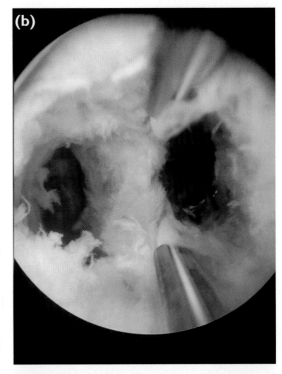

Figure 6.6. (a) Uterine septum (didelphis); (b) thick intra-uterine septum.

Recurrent miscarriage

Outpatient hysteroscopy is an ideal tool for diagnosing the structural anomalies that are associated with recurrent miscarriages.

Congenital anomalies of the uterus

Congenital anomalies associated with infertility include uterine didelphis, unicornuate and bicornuate uterus (Fig. 6.6a), and septate uterus (Fig. 6.6b). There is a high rate of spontaneous miscarriage and of preterm labour (between 25–47%) when these structural anomalies exist.

Other conditions associated with recurrent miscarriage diagnosed by outpatient hysteroscopy are uterine synechiae, uterine hypoplasia due to *in utero* exposure to diethylstilbestrol, and cervical canal anomalies. Although hysteroscopy is not useful in diagnosing cervical incompetence, it identifies cervical adhesions, atresia and polyps (Fig. 6.7). Cervical incompetence may be suspected

on withdrawal of the hysteroscope as a loss of anatomical relationship between the corpus and cervix and the disappearance of the sphincter-like action of the internal cervical os. The surgeon would also suspect cervical incompetence when the hysteroscope passes easily, the uterus

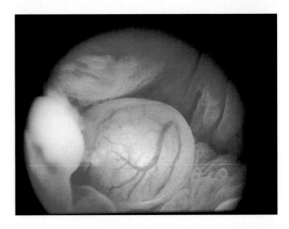

Figure 6.7. Endocervical polyp.

fails to distend, and there is loss of the liquid distension medium back through the cervix.

CONTRA-INDICATIONS TO AMBULATORY HYSTEROSCOPY

Absolute contra-indications

Cervical cancer

Hysteroscopy should not be performed in the presence of cervical carcinoma because of the danger of opening blood or lymphatic vessels and causing systemic dissemination of malignant cells.

Heavy uterine bleeding

Hysteroscopy should be avoided during menstruation because the view is usually unsatisfactory. There is also a theoretical risk of disseminating endometrial cells into the pelvis and causing endometriosis. Moderate uterine bleeding does not prevent adequate visualisation of the endometrial cavity but heavy bleeding will prevent clear views regardless of the distension medium used and it will promote intravasation of the distension medium. Despite this, there have been reports of hysteroscopy being performed during persistent heavy bleeding. In this situation, the only effective instrument is a double-channel, continuous flow hysteroscope. The pressure of the distension fluid will often arrest the bleeding and allow the residual blood to be flushed out.

Pelvic inflammatory disease

This is an absolute contra-indication to hysteroscopy because of the danger of causing extended, ascending infection and peritonitis. The procedure should be delayed until the infection has been eradicated. The only exception is a 'lost' IUCD-associated infection where hysteroscopy may be necessary to locate and remove it. The procedure should be performed under antibiotic cover.

Relative contra-indications

Pregnancy

Pregnancy is generally considered a contra-indication to hysteroscopy but it may be necessary to perform hysteroscopy to remove an IUCD, or to diagnose retained products of conception where there has been persistent post-abortal bleeding. However, ultrasonography has replaced endoscopy in many such cases. The myometrium in the gravid uterus is much more distensible than in the non-pregnant organ which has a strong, resistant muscular wall. Uterine distension with gas can cause the uterus to distend like a balloon resulting in accumulation of carbon dioxide which may lead to separation of the placenta and retroplacental bleeding. The accumulated gas may then flow as a bolus into the ruptured uterine veins causing a massive gas embolus. It is important, therefore, that hysteroscopy in pregnancy is only performed by an expert surgeon who is aware of these possibilities and that the gas flow is restricted to 20 ml/min with an intra-uterine pressure of less than 50 mmHg. It is also important to remember that the optic nerve of the fetus may be damaged by the hysteroscope light after the tenth week of pregnancy, although there does not appear to be any danger before this stage.

Recent uterine perforation

The risk of repeat uterine perforation is considerably greater in such patients as the healing process may leave a weak scar.

Cervical stenosis

It may be necessary to proceed with extreme caution or, on occasions, simply decide not to attempt to perform the procedure as the risk of uterine perforation is considerably greater in such patients. The role of an experienced operator should not be underestimated in this situation (see Chapter 8).

Cardiorespiratory disease

In severe cardiorespiratory diseases, the use of carbon dioxide as the distension medium may cause gas embolism. The risk has probably been under-reported because of the high solubility of carbon dioxide and the consequent difficulty in substantiating the diagnosis.

Uncooperative patient

Inability to tolerate a speculum can be a relative contra-indication, but this can be overcome using the vaginoscopic technique.

Inexperienced surgeon

Key points

➢ Abnormal uterine bleeding is the commonest reason for hysteroscopic examination.

➢ Endometrial carcinoma is rare before the age of 40 years and its incidence rises steeply between ages 45–55 years. Between 5–10% of all women with postmenopausal bleeding will have endometrial cancer or precancerous lesions.

➢ Structural lesions responsible for abnormal uterine bleeding are often at their peak during the perimenopausal period; these include focal lesions like endometrial polyps and submucous fibroids and diffuse lesions like endometrial atrophy, hyperplasia, cancer and diffuse adenomyosis.

➢ Blind dilatation and curettage only samples 60% of the endometrium; most focal lesions (polyps and fibroids) which will be obvious at hysteroscopy are missed by dilatation and curettage.

➢ Hysteroscopy is not used routinely in the investigation of infertility.

➢ The main indication for use of hysteroscopy in the investigation of infertility is in clarifying intra-uterine status when an abnormal hysterosalpingograaphy result is obtained.

MULTIPLE CHOICE QUESTIONS

1. **Indications for outpatient hysteroscopy include:**

    Resection of type II submucous fibroids   True/False

    Diagnosis of uterine synechiae   True/False

    Location and retrieval of lost or misplaced intrauterine contraceptive device   True/False

    Transcervical resection of the endometrium for menorrhagia   True/False

2. **Abnormal uterine bleeding:**

    Is the commonest reason for hysteroscopic examination   True/False

Abnormal uterine bleeding accounts for more than 50% of referrals to the gynaecologist	True/False
Structural lesions responsible for abnormal uterine bleeding are often at their peak during the postmenopausal period	True/False
Between 5–10% of all women with postmenopausal bleeding will have endometrial cancer	True/False

3. In the investigation of infertility:

Outpatient hysteroscopy is used routinely	True/False
Hysteroscopy has a high false-positive rate due to distortion of the uterine cavity from mucus, debris, and blood	True/False
Outpatient hysteroscopy is the diagnostic procedure of choice in diagnosing intra-uterine anomalies in infertile patients	True/False
Outpatient hysteroscopy has a sensitivity of 85% in detecting tubal pathology	True/False

4. In infertility:

Of women presenting with infertility, 20% have endometrial polyps	True/False
There is good evidence that women with polyps have a higher rate of spontaneous miscarriage	True/False
The value of routine hysteroscopic removal of these polyps before fertility treatment is unknown	True/False
There is evidence to show that fibroids directly affect fertility	True/False

5. Absolute contra-indications to outpatient hysteroscopy include:

Recent uterine perforation	True/False
Pregnancy	True/False
Cervical cancer	True/False
Heavy uterine bleeding	True/False

7 Indications for ambulatory operative hysteroscopy

OBJECTIVE: To give an overview of the indications for ambulatory operative hysteroscopic procedures.

CONTENTS
Targeted biopsy
Endocervical and endometrial polypectomy
Treatment of submucous fibroids
Division of intra-uterine adhesions
Division of uterine septa

Removal of 'lost' IUDs
Outpatient hysteroscopic sterilisation Essure™
Outpatient endometrial ablation
Key points
MCQs

Improvements in the last decade in design and the manufacturing of smaller diameter hysteroscopes have made it possible to carry out operative hysteroscopy in the outpatient setting without the need for cervical dilatation or anaesthesia in most cases. These instruments have an outer sheath diameter of < 5 mm and incorporate working channels and continuous flow features. Other advances include the use of bipolar energy rather than monopolar energy thus making it possible to use normal saline rather than non-ionic distension media (glycine, sorbitol, and mannitol).These advances have made ambulatory operative hysteroscopy a time-efficient and cost-effective, safe procedure.

TARGETED BIOPSY

Focal lesions in the endometrium, which are suspicious or look abnormal, are best biopsied using a targeted approach. Providing the hysteroscope has an operative channel then the surgeon can, under direct vision, take tissue samples from the area. The hysteroscopist can use a biopsy cup or grasping forceps passed down the operating channel. For outpatient hysteroscopy, the operating channel is usually 5–7 Fr.

ENDOCERVICAL AND ENDOMETRIAL POLYPECTOMY

Polyps on the ectocervix can be removed by avulsion if they are pedunculated or using a LLETZ loop if they are sessile. This is best done after the hysteroscopy is completed to prevent any bleeding obscuring vision. If the polyp is in the endocervical canal then it is removed using the same technique as described below for endometrial polyps.

Endometrial polyps are proliferation and hypertrophy of the basal layer of the endometrium.

At hysteroscopy, they are smooth and soft, indenting easily on contact, the surface may oscillate in the current produced by the distension medium, and often have very little vascularisation. They are either sessile or pedunculated (see Fig. 6.3a–c). They can be removed by using:

- Mechanical instruments, *e.g.* snares, scissors or graspers passed down a 5–7 Fr operating channel under direct vision

- Bipolar electrodes in normal saline. A twizzle electrode (Fig. 3.9) can be used to slice a polyp into small segments that can then be retrieved by grasping forceps under direct vision. The authors would recommend removing the pieces at the end of the procedure. Removing each piece as it is separated can over dilate the cervix and produce loss of distension and vision. A spring electrode can be used to destroy the polyp by ablating the tissue. The disadvantage of this method is that there is no histology. Most experts would recommend that polyps of < 3 cm in diameter can be removed this way. This can be achieved in less than 15 minutes and will be tolerated by most women. Larger polyps take longer and are best managed by resection under general or regional anaesthesia.

TREATMENT OF SUBMUCOUS FIBROIDS

Fibroids are benign tumours composed of smooth muscle and fibrotic connective tissue. They affect 30% of women in their reproductive years and are a common finding at hysteroscopy for abnormal uterine bleeding (Fig. 6.4a,c). When seen at hysteroscopy, they show a superficial vascularisation through a thin endometrium as well as the whitish aspect of the myoma tissue, as compared with the surrounding endometrium and myometrium. They feel firm and cannot be indented easily with the hysteroscope or mechanical instruments and often distort the symmetry of

the uterine cavity. They can be classified as (Fig. 6.4a):

- Type 0: 100% of the fibroid is within the endometrial cavity

- Type I: > 50% is within the uterine cavity.

- Type II: < 50% is within the uterine cavity.

Most experts would recommend that only types 0 and I submucous fibroids of < 2 cm in diameter should be treated in the outpatient setting. They can be treated using:

- Mechanical instruments, *i.e.* scissors, to dissect them free or grasping forceps for the small type 0 submucous fibroids

- Bipolar instruments in normal saline. The spring electrode (Fig. 3.9) is particularly useful in ablating the fibroid tissue and returning the uterine cavity to a normal configuration.

DIVISION OF INTRA-UTERINE ADHESIONS

Intra-uterine adhesions result from trauma in the postpartum or post abortal period. It generally leads to hypmenorrhoea or amenorrhoea. Hysteroscopy is effective in evaluating the uterine cavity and outlining the precise distortion that exists from the adhesions and also permitting direct treatment. The extent of the adhesions varies from focal to multiple areas. The extent also determines the prognosis. Adhesions are classified as mild, moderate or severe. When mild, they are filmy, thin and usually only of recent occurrence, and are easily amenable to outpatient hysteroscopic division either by mechanical instruments or by bipolar electrosurgical methods. They have a better prognosis than the moderate or severe varieties. Moderate adhesions are fibromuscular, thick and covered by endometrium and may bleed on division. Severe adhesions are usually composed of connective tissue only, without endometrial covering and are unlikely to bleed on division as they are more fibrotic. Division of moderate and severe forms often requires general anaesthesia and concomitant laparoscopy.

In the outpatient setting, scissors or a twizzle electrode are used for division of mild to moderate adhesions under hysteroscopic vision. Of these patients, 90% have normal menstruation following treatment and 60–70% pregnancy rates occur depending on the severity before treatment (Fig.6.5a–f).

DIVISION OF UTERINE SEPTA

Of women with a septate uterus, 25% have recurrent pregnancy loss. The septa are poorly vascularised making them ideal for hystero-scopic division. Traditionally, division has been via the abdominal route entailing a laparotomy and uterotomy.

Hysteroscopic methods used for division are scissors, resectoscopes, cutting electrodes, fibre-optic laser and, more recently, the bipolar operating electrode. This offers the advantage of using saline (isotonic) fluid as the distension medium. Hystero-scopic division with scissors suffices for thin septum while thicker and broader ones may require a cutting electrode (e.g. twizzle electrode) or the use of a resectoscope under general or regional anaesthesia (Fig. 7.1a,b). Every effort should be made to ensure a thick covering of myometrium at the uterine fundus (transvaginal scan). If this is not certain then the division is best carried out under laparoscopic control to maintain uniform transillumination of the fundal portion of the uterus while the septum is divided.

Hysteroscopic division: (i) offers high success rates; (ii) avoids the increased morbidity from an abdominal operation; (iii) is more cost effective; and (iv) avoids the risk of postoperative intra-abdominal adhesions.

Following hysteroscopic division, successful pregnancy rates of 85–90% have been quoted in some series. Generally, patients are advised to

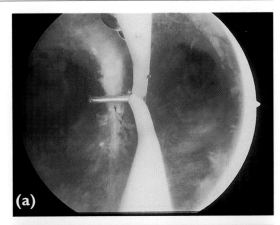

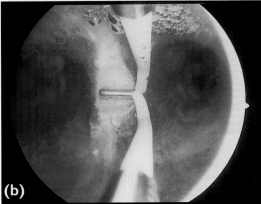

Figure 7.1 (**a** and **b**) Division of partial uterine septum.

delay pregnancy for at least 4–6 weeks. Caesarean section is not mandatory should pregnancy be carried to term.

REMOVAL OF 'LOST' IUDS

In the majority of cases of 'lost' IUDs, the device is still present in the uterine cavity with its thread curled up into the uterine cavity out of view on speculum examination. Pelvic ultrasound scan will locate the IUD and confirm its presence inside the cavity. If there is doubt, a plain abdominal X-ray should be ordered.

Hysteroscopy is invaluable in the removal of the IUD from the uterus. This can be carried out in the outpatient setting. A hysteroscope with an opera-

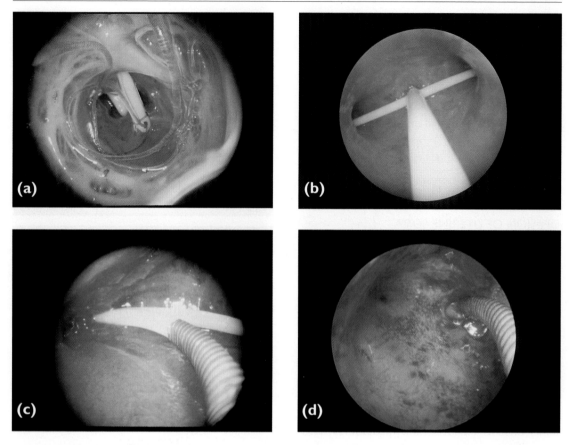

Figure 7.2 (a) Intrauterine contraceptive device or IUD; (b) IUD in uterus; (c) removal of IUD; (d) hysteroscopic view of partially embedded IUD.

tive channel is used with grasping forceps inserted into the uterus and either the thread or the IUD itself is grasped with the forceps and the hysteroscope is withdrawn together with the IUD (Fig. 7.2).

OUTPATIENT HYSTEROSCOPIC STERILISATION (ESSURE™)

Hysteroscopic sterilisation performed in an outpatient setting aims to reduce the risks from a general anaesthesia, reduce the morbidity associated with having an abdominal incision, has a shorter recovery period and aims to be more cost effective than other methods of permanent contraception.

A new method that tries to achieve this is the Essure™ permanent contraceptive system developed by Conceptus Inc. The Essure™ system consists of the Essure™ micro-insert, a disposable delivery system, and a disposable split introducer. A standard hysteroscope with a 5-Fr working channel, continuous flow, and a 12–30° angled lens is used when sterilising with Essure™.

The Essure™ micro-insert consists of a stainless steel inner coil, a nitinol, super-elastic outer coil, and polyethylene (PET) fibres. The PET fibres are wound in and around the inner coil. The micro-insert is 4 cm in length and 0.8 mm in diameter in its wound-down configuration. When released, the outer coil expands to 1.5–2.0 mm to

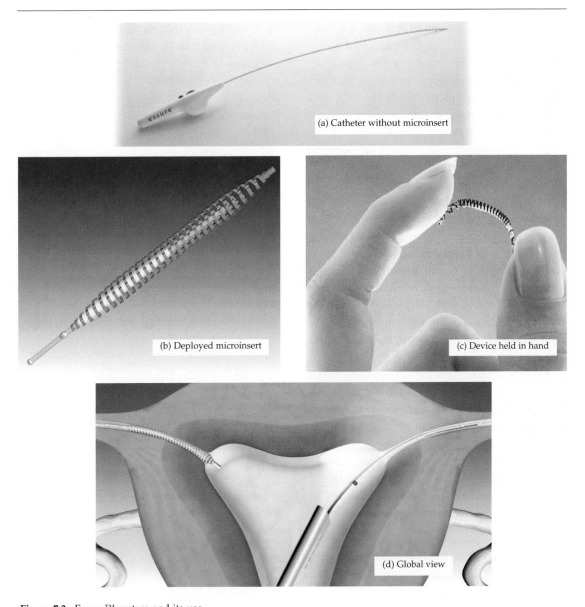

(a) Catheter without microinsert

(b) Deployed microinsert

(c) Device held in hand

(d) Global view

Figure 7.3 Essure™ system and its use.

anchor the micro-insert in the varied diameters and shapes of any Fallopian tube (Fig. 7.3).

The Essure™ micro-insert remains anchored in the Fallopian tube, placed across the utero–tubal junction. The diameter of the micro-insert is larger trailing into the uterus than within the tubal lumen. This difference in the diameters is intended to prevent migration toward the peritoneal cav-

ity. The PET fibres elicit tissue in-growth. The PET fibre mesh and the micro-insert act as scaffolding into which the tissue grows, anchoring the micro-insert within the fallopian tube and occluding the tube, resulting in sterilisation.

A strong fibrous tissue response occurs with histological evidence of both loose and dense smooth muscle cells migrating from the fallopian tube wall into the space between the inner and outer coil (Fig. 7.5d). This response is consistent in all patients over 3 months.

The disposable delivery system consists of a single-handed ergonomic handle, which contains a delivery wire, release catheter, delivery catheter, and micro-insert.

The ergonomic handle controls delivery and release (Fig. 7.3a). A thumbwheel on the handle allows the hysteroscopist to retract both the delivery catheter and the release catheter. The delivery wire is detached from the micro-insert by rotating the system. The split introducer helps protect the micro-insert as it passes through the port of the working channel of the hysteroscope. The proximal end of the micro-inset is evaluated by hysteroscopy to ensure that 5–10 mm (5–8 coils) of trailing micro-insert are in the uterine cavity. The same procedure is carried out in the opposite fallopian tube (Figs 7.4 and 7.5).

In early studies, bilateral tubal occlusion was demonstrated in 96% of cases and 6-months' follow-up confirmed bilateral occlusion in all patients. Essure™ is 99.80% effective in preventing pregnancy after 3 years of follow-up. It can be performed in 15 to 30 minutes and has a high patient satisfaction rating. Bilateral placement rate occurs in 86% (first attempt) and 90% (with second attempt). An alternative method of contraception must be used for 3 months after the procedure. Results of a pivotal study of adverse or other events that delayed or prevented reliance on Essure™ for contraception are summarised in Table 7.1. The manufacturers advise an X-ray or ultrasound scan to check the correct placement of the microinserts at 3 months.

OUTPATIENT ENDOMETRIAL ABLATION

Endometrial ablation is designed to treat abnormal uterine bleeding in women with no intra-uterine pathology. The ablative devices more suited for the outpatient setting are the second generation, so called, global endometrial ablation devices. There have been many innovative devices proposed for achieving rapid, simple global endometrial ablation. The types of energy sources include hot water, cryocautery, microwave, laser, and radio-frequency energy. These procedures can be done in an outpatient setting using local anaesthetic. In the future, newer devices will undoubtedly be approved.

Balloon devices

There are two balloons in clinical use, which use a combination of heating and pressure to achieve

Table 7.1. Adverse or other events that delay or prevent reliance on Essure™ for contraception

Event	Number	Percentage
Expulsion	14/476	2.9%*
Perforation	5/476	1.1%
Unsatisfactory micro-insert location	3/476	0.6%
Initial tubal patency	16/456	3.5%**

* Fourteen women experienced an expulsion; however, 9 of these 14 women chose to undergo a second micro-insert placement procedure, which was successful in all 9 cases.

** Tubal patency was demonstrated in 16 women at the 3-month HSG, but all 16 women were shown to have tubal occlusion at a repeat HSG performed 6–7 months after Essure™ placement.

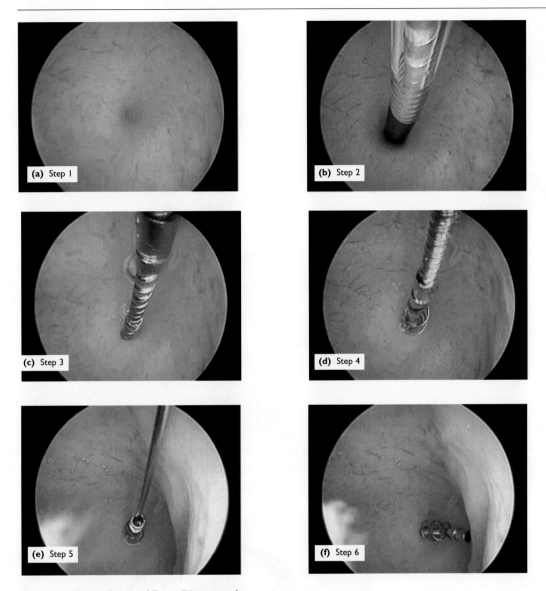

Figure 7.4 Internal view of Essure™ system placement.

endometrial destruction. They are only used in regular cavities, so 30% of women with menstrual problems would be excluded from treatment with these devices. Cavity size is also limited to between 4–10 cm. They cause pain by uterine distension during treatment under local anaesthetic. Most authors suggest full doses of non-steroidal anti-inflammatory drugs prior to treatment and rescue

analgesia if needed (nitrous oxide or paracervical block). Neither require endometrial priming.

Thermachoice system

The Thermachoice system (a product of GyneCare) is a closed system using a sculptured silicone balloon. Its external diameter is 4.5 mm, so rarely needs cervical dilatation prior to insertion. The

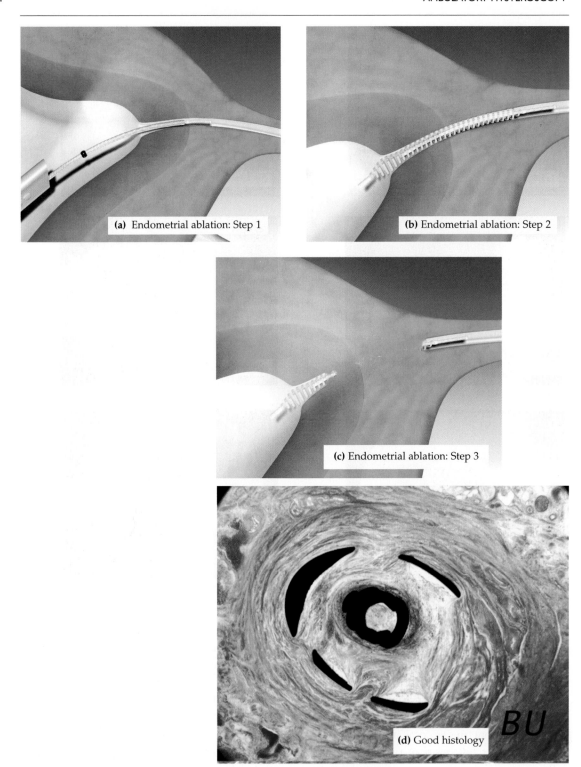

Figure 7.5   Essure™ system placement and histological effects.

device is inserted into the uterus and expanded to pressures of between 160–180 mmHg using sterile dextrose 5%. A microprocessor controls heating to 87°C. Once treatment temperature is reached, the treatment time is 8 minutes. The whole procedure usually takes 15 minutes. One-year patient satisfaction rates are 85% with 15–23% amenorrhoea rates (Fig. 7.6).

Cavatern

This is a similar device to Thermachoice but the silicone balloon is inflated to 180–200 mm Hg with a

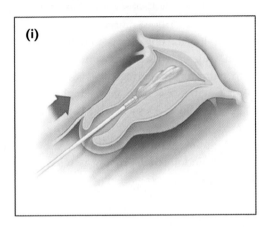
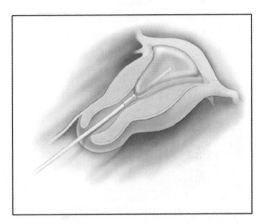
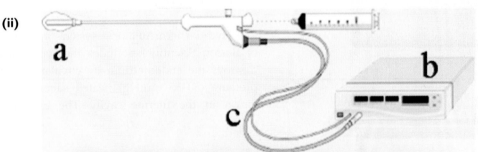
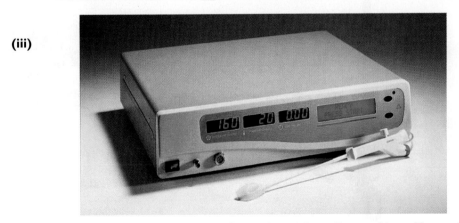

Figure 7.6 Thermachoice system: (**a**) single use balloon catheter, 4–5 mm diameter; (**b**) reusable controller; (**c**) umbilical cable and power cable.

treatment temperature of 75°C for 15 minutes. The device has an external diameter of 8 mm, so requires cervical dilatation before insertion. Cavaterm is not used frequently in the outpatient setting in the UK.

Microwave endometrial ablation

The microwave endometrial ablation device (a product of Microsulis) uses a software-controlled unit with microwave energy at a fixed frequency of 9.2 GHz. The operating power is 42 W. The microwave energy is delivered by an 8-mm

diameter probe, which heats the tissue to 80–90°C. This gives reliable tissue destruction to 4–5 mm depth. It is performed under local anaesthetic but the cervix needs dilating to Hegar 9 prior to insertion, so 4-quadrant cervical block is recommended. However, there is no uterine distension and treatment time is short – 3 minutes in a normal sized cavity. Patient satisfaction rate at 1 year is 87% and amenorrhoea rates of 33–53% have been reported. It is the only device initially licensed for use in patients with submucous fibroids up to 3 cm diameter or uterine cavity depth of up to 14 cm. Cavities of > 11 cm have a higher chance of treatment failure. Women who have had lower segment caesarean section can be treated providing the scar thickness measured by TVS is > 8 mm. Endometrial priming is recommended (Fig. 7.7a,b).

Hydro ThermAblator™

The Hydro ThermAblator™ system (a product of Boston Scientific) occludes the cervix and destroys the endometrium by circulating low pressure (50–55 mmHg) heated saline under vision in the uterine cavity. The insulated,

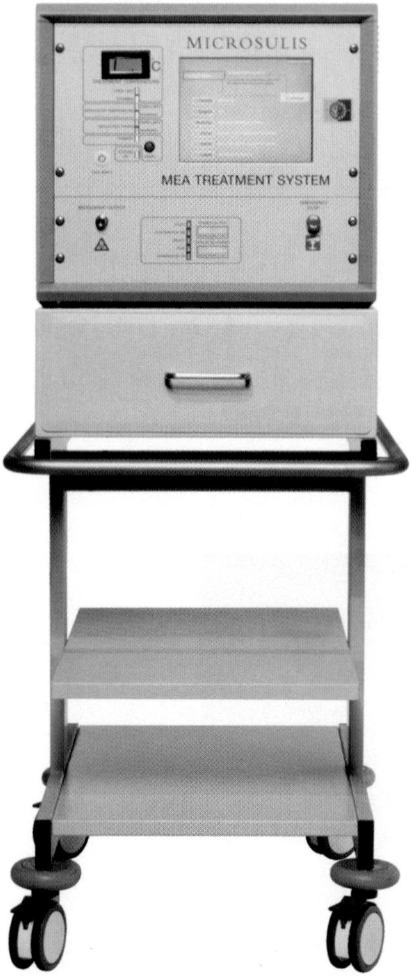

(a)

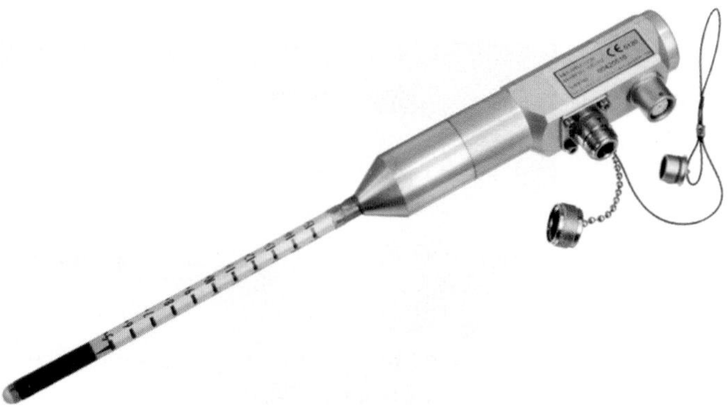

(b)

Figure 7.7 Microwave endometrial ablation system.

disposable sheath is 7.8 mm in diameter and fits over most commercially available 3-mm hysteroscopes. The cervix needs dilatation to Hegar 8 to allow insertion of the device. The uterine cavity should measure < 12 cm but cavities with fibroids can be treated. It takes 3 minutes to heat the saline to the treatment temperature of 90°C. The treatment time is then 10 minutes followed by a cooling period of a further minute before the device can be withdrawn. The heated saline thus bathes the endometrial cavity with the cervix sealed. If more than 10 ml of fluid is lost, the system shuts down. There is a theoretical possibility of leakage of heated saline into the vagina causing burns but because of the fail-safe shut-down system this is extremely unlikely. Because of the low pressures used (lower than the 60 mm opening pressure of the tubal ostia), fluid spillage into the peritoneal cavity does not occur. It has been performed under local anaesthesia using para-cervical block but the procedure time of 15 minutes makes treatment in the outpatient setting less appealing to the patient. One-year success rate is 94% with reported amenorrhoea rates of 40–60%. Endometrial priming is recommended (Fig. 7.8).

NovaSure

NovaSure (a product of Cytec) is a disposable, impedance-controlled device. No endometrial priming is needed. .It uses bipolar energy delivered through a gold-plated mesh mounted on a flexible frame, which conforms to the shape of the uterine cavity. The device is 6.9 mm in diameter and so requires cervical dilatation. Regular cavities between 6–11 cm can be treated with this device. Cavity integrity is checked using a small amount of CO_2. Once the device is seated, it vaporises the endometrium regardless of thickness using bipolar energy. As tissue destruction continues, the resistance to flow of current increases until tissue impedance reaches

50 ohms. Treatment time is calculated by the generator based on tissue impedance. Once impedance reaches 50 ohms or treatment time reaches 2 minutes, the treatment is complete. Procedure time has been reported at 5 minutes, which includes treatment time and time for placing the device. There is no uterine distension. The amenorrhoea rate at 1 year is 43% with a success rate of 90%.

Other devices

Cryoablation: HerOption

HerOption uses tissue freezing to destroy the endometrium by causing tissue necrosis. It seems to produce less scarring than heat. Priming is at the surgeon's discretion. It uses a disposable 5.5-mm freezing probe, which is inserted into the uterus under ultrasound guidance. The company recommends paracervical block but also states that the auto-anaesthetic effects of freezing decrease the pain of the procedure and post-procedure cramping. The probe is inserted first into one cornua and the freeze cycle initiated. Once the ice ball reaches within 2–3 mm of the serosal surface (4–6 minutes), as seen on ultrasound, the thaw cycle is started. Once thawed, the probe is moved to the other cornua and the process repeated (the second freeze is usually 6 minutes). The process, therefore, needs two freeze-thaw cycles. One-year success rates are 94% and amenorrhoea rate is 30%.

Endometrial laser intra-uterine thermotherapy (ELITT)

ELITT uses laser light at 830-nm wavelength to destroy the endometrium by heating. The device is a disposable, multiple laser-fibre hand-piece which does not need to be in contact with the endo-metrium to have its effect. The laser light is diffused inside the uterine cavity in all directions and reaches even the most inaccessible areas. The hand-piece is 7 mm in diameter so the cervix has to be dilated prior to insertion. Once deployed in the

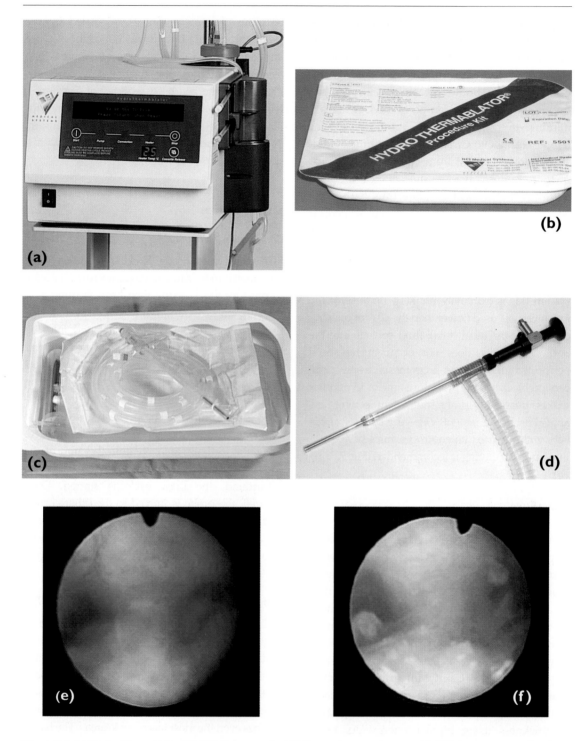

Figure 7.8 (a) Hydro ThermAblator™ (HTA) system; (b,c) HTA system procedure set; (d) HTA hysteroscopic sheath; (e) pretreatment; (f) post-treatment.

uterine cavity, the laser is activated for a 7-minute treatment cycle. The device is then closed and removed from the uterus. Initial results indicate that the success rate at 1 year is 86% with an amenorrhoea rate of 70%. Endometrial priming is recommended.

Key points

➤ Improvements in the last decade in the design and manufacturing of smaller diameter hysteroscopes (< 5 mm) have made it possible to carry out operative hysteroscopy in the outpatient setting without the need for cervical dilatation or anaesthesia in most cases.

➤ Other advances include the use of bipolar energy rather than monopolar energy thus making it possible to use normal saline rather than non-ionic distension media (glycine, sorbitol, and mannitol).

➤ Most experts recommend that only type 0 and type I submucous fibroids of < 2 cm in diameter should be treated in the outpatient setting.

➤ Mild, intra-uterine adhesions are easily amenable to outpatient hysteroscopic division. Division of the moderate and severe forms often requires general anaesthesia and concomitant laparoscopy.

➤ Uterine septa are usually poorly vascularised making them ideal for hysteroscopic division.

➤ In the majority of cases of 'lost' IUDs, the device is still present in the uterine cavity with its thread curled up into the uterine cavity out of view on speculum examination. This can be easily retrieved with outpatient hysteroscopy.

➤ Essure™ is a new system designed to achieve permanent contraception via outpatient hysteroscopic sterilisation.

➤ The ablative devices more suited for the outpatient setting using local anaesthetic are the second generation, so called, global endometrial ablation devices.

➤ The microwave endometrial ablation device may be used in patients with submucous fibroids up to 3 cm in diameter or a uterine cavity depth of up to 14 cm.

MULTIPLE CHOICE QUESTIONS

1. **Indications for ambulatory operative hysteroscopy**

    Targeted biopsy under direct vision — True/False

    Most experts would recommend that polyps of up to 5 cm in diameter can be removed — True/False

    Most experts would recommend that type 0, type I and type II submucous fibroids can all be treated in the outpatient setting — True/False

    In the majority of cases of lost IUDs, the device is still present in the uterine cavity — True/False

2. **Intra-uterine adhesions**

    Result from trauma in the postpartum or post-abortal period   True/False

    Generally lead to menorrhagia   True/False

    Moderate adhesions are fibromuscular, thick and avascular   True/False

    Severe adhesions are likely to bleed on division   True/False

3. **Division of uterine septa**

    25% of women with a septate uterus have recurrent pregnancy loss   True/False

    The septa are poorly vascularised making them ideal for hysteroscopic division   True/False

    Hysteroscopic division yields low success rates   True/False

    Caesarean section is mandatory should pregnancy be carried to term   True/False

4. **Outpatient endometrial ablation**

    The approved devices have patient satisfaction rates of more than 80%   True/False

    With microwave endometrial ablation (MEA) failure is more likely to occur when the uterine cavity is greater than 12 cm   True/False

    MEA can be used when intra-uterine fibroids exist   True/False

    Endometrial priming is an absolute requirement   True/False

5. **Essure™**

    Essure™ hysteroscopic sterilisation is 99.8% effective in preventing pregnancy after 3 years' follow-up   True/False

    It takes over 45 minutes to perform   True/False

    Has a high patient satisfaction rating   True/False

    An alternative method of contraception must be used for 3 months after the procedure   True/False

8 Complications of diagnostic and operative ambulatory hysteroscopy

OBJECTIVE: To provide a detailed overview of possible complications of hysteroscopy in the ambulatory setting, both minor and major.

CONTENTS
Complications of positioning the patient
Complications of excessive absorption of distendion media
Complications of diagnostic hysteroscopy in the ambulatory setting
Complications of operative hysteroscopy in the ambulatory setting
Failure of resolution of the presenting symptoms
Failure to make an accurate diagnosis
Avoidance of complications
Key points
MCQs

Ambulatory hysteroscopy is a safe procedure by any imaginable standard. Complications can occur when inappropriate instruments or techniques are used (Table 8.1). Most complications of hysteroscopy are rare and if they do occur, they are seldom life-threatening particularly in diagnostic procedures. A recent UK Royal College of Obstetricians and Gynaecologists' guideline for taking consent for diagnostic hysteroscopy under general anaesthetic quoted a figure as low as 8/1000 for uterine perforation. For ambulatory procedures, the figure is much lower. In a large systematic review of studies of over 25,000 women, only eight (3/10,000) cases of potentially serious complications (pelvic infection, uterine perforations [4], bladder perforation, and precipitation of a hypocalcaemic crisis and an anginal episode) were reported. Operative hysteroscopic procedures are more risky, with uterine perforation being the most common complication. However, hysteroscopic polypectomy is associated with lower rates of complications (12 times lower than synechiolysis). Some of the complications are entry-related, so avoid dilating the cervix unnecessarily and always introduce the hysteroscope under direct vision. Other complications are related to surgeons' experience and type of procedure. Among other hysteroscopic procedures, resection of fibroids and uterine septa have significantly higher rates of complications (4–7 times higher operative complications than polypectomy) mainly due to fluid intravasation. Ambulatory operative procedures tend to be short in duration; as the patient is awake and responsive to painful stimuli, the chances are that fluid intravasation problems are unlikely and difficult procedure will be abandoned early due to patient intolerance minimising the risk of complications.

COMPLICATIONS OF POSITIONING THE PATIENT

Correct position

Positioning the patient is important to prevent musculoskeletal and neurological complications. As explained in Chapter 4, hysteroscopy is performed using the colposcopy couch in the lithotomy position with legs apart supported by leg rests with the buttocks a few centimetres extending beyond the end of the table (after the foot of the table is lowered or removed). The back should be flat on the table not flexed to avoid postoperative lower back discomfort. No joint in the leg is flexed over 60° to avoid femoral nerve compression (associated with extreme flexion, abduction, and lateral rotation at the hip).

Table 8.1. Complications of diagnostic and operative ambulatory hysteroscopy

Complications of positioning the patient
> Correct position
> Damage to soft tissues
> Nerve injuries
> Deep venous thrombosis

Complications of excessive absorption of distendion media
> Carbon dioxide
> Fluids

Complications of diagnostic hysteroscopy in the ambulatory setting
> Uterine perforation
> Vaso-vagal reflex
> Heavy bleeding
> Abnormal discharge
> Fever

Complications of operative hysteroscopy in the ambulatory setting
> Intra-operative complications
> > 1. Vaso-vagal reflex
> > 2. Cervical trauma
> > 3. Uterine perforation
> > 4. Haemorrhage

> Delayed complications
> > 1. Infection
> > 2. Vaginal discharge
> > 3. Adhesion formation

Failure of resolution of the presenting symptoms

Failure to make an accurate diagnosis

Avoiding excessive pressure on the lateral aspect of the lower legs within the stirrups helps avoid perineal nerve compression and 'foot drop'.

Incorrect positioning may result in:

Damage to soft tissues

It is the responsibility of the surgeon to ensure that there is no injury from moving parts of the table to the patient's soft tissues. As bipolar energy is the main energy source used in ambulatory setting, patient safety concerns related to monopolar energy (i.e. to ensure that no part of the patient is in contact with metal parts of the table because these can act as return plates for electrical energy and burns can occur at the point of contact) is not applicable.

Nerve injuries

Injury can result after 15 minutes in the wrong position. Pressure on the perineal nerve from lithotomy poles may result in paraesthesia and foot drop. Since patients are awake, they should be instructed to lift their legs and place them apart in the supports. Extra care should be given to patients with a prosthesis or prior joint surgery.

Deep venous thrombosis

This can result from prolonged compression of the calves by the leg supports. The surgeon should ensure that the calves are adequately supported and well padded if the patient is undergoing a long outpatient procedure. In high-risk cases, stocking may be considered.

COMPLICATIONS OF EXCESSIVE ABSORPTION OF DISTENSION MEDIA

Complications produced by the distension media are specific to hysteroscopic surgery though they also occur in endoscopic prostatic procedures. The problems are less likely in ambulatory procedures, but are detailed here for completeness. It is essential that all operating room staff are familiar with the side-effects of the absorption of distension media and that the responsibility for fluid balance is taken by a designated member of staff.

The nature of the complications depends on the type of medium in use, which may be gaseous (e.g. carbon dioxide) or fluid and depends on whether the fluid is of high or low viscosity.

Carbon dioxide

Cardiac arrhythmia can occur even with diagnostic hysteroscopy using CO_2. The complication should be extremely rare if the correct insufflator is used. The hysteroflator delivers CO_2 at a rate of not more than 100 ml/min whereas the laparoflator can deliver 1–6 litres in the same time. A laparoflator should NEVER be used for hysteroscopy. It is rare for CO_2 to produce any side-effects if gas embolism of less than 400 ml occurs. Gas embolism during hysteroscopy is rare but can sometimes be rapidly fatal. Symptomatic gas embolism can occur when undissolved gas (air, CO_2) accumulates in the heart and/or pulmonary arteries compromising circulation and causing serious shock or death. Suspicion should arise when the patient suddenly gasps for air, with impalpable pulse, tonic convulsions, consciousness loss and cardiac arrest. Heart sounds suggesting intracardiac gas may be heard (mill-wheel murmur). The importance of monitoring to aid a rapid diagnosis and immediate treatment remarkably improves the outcome. Immediate cardiopulmonary resuscitation is required until the crash team arrives and the patient is admitted to the intensive care unit. The diagnosis may be confirmed by aspiration of foamy blood from the central venous line, which is diagnostic and therapeutic at the same time.

Fluids

Accurate fluid balance is mandatory in any operative hysteroscopic procedure. The severity and management of fluid overload depends on the nature of the medium in use and on the volume used. If such complications should occur during the procedure, surgery must be abandoned. Most surgeons would be concerned at 750 ml deficit and would end the procedure at 1000 ml. Table 8.2 summarises the available fluid distension media and their side effects.

Electrolytic solutions (normal saline, lactated Ringer's) are capable of conducting electricity; therefore, cannot be used in conjunction with monopolar energy but can be used in diagnostic hysteroscopy and in operative cases in which mechanical instruments, laser or bipolar energy are used.

Non-electrolytic solutions (glycine 1.5%, mannitol 5%) eliminate problems with electrical

---

Table 8.2 Fluid distension media used in hysteroscopy

Electrolytic solutions are capable of conducting electricity; therefore, cannot be used in conjunction with monopolar electrosurgical devices. Normal saline and Lactated Ringer's are recommended by the American Association of Gynecologic Laparoscopists (AAGL) for use in diagnostic cases and in operative cases in which mechanical instruments, laser or bipolar energy are used

• **Normal saline**	Used for diagnostic hysteroscopy, operative procedures utilising lasers, mechanical instruments or bipolar electrosurgical devices. Saline overload produces a simple hypervolaemic state which may be treated by insertion of a central venous line, administration of a diuretic, oxygen and, if necessary, cardiac stimulants. A blood pressure cuff may be applied to each limb in rotation to occlude venous return, which, in effect, performs a bloodless phlebotomy

Non-electrolytic solutions eliminate problems with electrical conductivity, but can increase the risk to patients of hyponatraemia and other complications

• **Water**	Used until the late 1980s, but problems with water intoxication and haemolysis have discontinued its use
• **Glucose**	Contra-indicated in glucose-intolerant patients
• **Glycine 1.5%**	Used in conjunction with monopolar electrosurgical energy. Metabolises into ammonia, which can cross the blood brain barrier, causing agitation, dizziness, vomiting and coma. Glycine is the commonest fluid in use in UK practice
• **Mannitol 5%**	Has a diuretic effect, can cause hypotension and circulatory collapse. Recommended by AAGL instead of glycine or sorbitol when using monopolar energy
• **Dextran**	Complications include coagulation disorders, allergic reactions and adult respiratory distress syndrome
• **Sorbitol**	Metabolises to fructose in the liver. Should not be used in fructose-intolerant patients

conductivity and can be used in conjunction with monopolar energy, but can increase the risk to patients of hyponatraemia and other complications.

Prevention of fluid overload

The above complications usually occur in the immediate postoperative period. Prevention can be accomplished by:

1. Using appropriate distension media and delivery systems.

2. Keeping operating times to a minimum.

3. Keeping fluid pressures as low as possible because fluid absorption occurs if it exceeds venous pressure.

4. Meticulous fluid balance. The procedure must be abandoned if the deficit rises to 750–1000 ml.

Treatment of fluid overload

The treatment of fluid overload depends largely on the type of distension fluid used during hysteroscopy. Fluid overload rarely occurs during procedures in which electrolyte-containing fluid such as normal saline or lactated Ringer's is used. When excessive intravasation with isotonic solution combinations such as 5% mannitol or a mannitol/sorbitol mixture occurs, no specific treatment may be necessary as these fluids have a diuretic effect which rids the body of excess fluid. If the patient is healthy and the sodium levels are not extremely low, fluid restriction and observation should be sufficient as the patient diureses. Since hypokalaemia and hypocalcaemia can often occur in conjunction with hyponatraemia, serum potassium and calcium levels should be monitored and replacement provided as necessary. Hyponatraemia can cause adverse neurological and cardiovascular effects such as muscle twitching and weakness, seizures, hypotension, and tachycardia.

The administration of hypertonic saline may not be necessary unless such neuromuscular or cardiac abnormalities occur.

Hyponatraemia caused by excessive intravasation of non-electrolyte distension media has more serious adverse effects and requires more complex treatment. Patients suffering from hyponatraemia resulting from the intravasation of a hypotonic fluid are at risk of hypotension, pulmonary oedema, cerebral oedema, and cardiovascular collapse. Any patient with a serum sodium level less than 120 mEq/l due to the absorption of glycine, sorbitol, or other hypotonic fluid should be monitored and treated in a critical-care setting. Treatment is with 3% sodium chloride sufficient to raise the serum sodium level by about 1 mEq/l. Correction to more than 135 mEq/l may result in adverse cerebral effects. The administration of diuretics may also be necessary. Although most women recover, seizures, permanent brain damage, and death have been reported.

COMPLICATIONS OF DIAGNOSTIC HYSTEROSCOPY IN THE AMBULATORY SETTING

Uterine perforation

Diagnostic hysteroscopy is a safe procedure that only rarely causes complications. Uterine perforation is a rare event. In the experience of the authors with a combined ten years of outpatient practice, there were only two cases in over 10,000 patients. As long as hysteroscopy is performed under vision at all times then perforation will not occur. Perforation will occur when the cervix is dilated in cases where there is cervical stenosis. Perforation occurs more frequently at the level of the fundus without significant bleeding. When perforation occurs, the woman will need admission, antibiotic cover and observation for signs of intraperitoneal bleeding. Laparoscopy should be performed only if there are concerns about intraperitoneal bleeding and antibiotics administered.

The other complications are:

(i) vaso-vagal reflex;

(ii) heavy bleeding;

(iii) abnormal discharge; and

(iv) fever over 38.3°C. The incidence of infection was reported as 2/1000 in over 4000 diagnostic hysteroscopies in one large cohort study.

COMPLICATIONS OF OPERATIVE HYSTEROSCOPY IN THE AMBULATORY SETTING

Complications of the procedure may arise during the operation or be delayed. Intra-operative complications include uterine perforation, cervical trauma and haemorrhage. Late-onset complications include infection, discharge and adhesion formation.

Intra-operative complications

Vaso-vagal reflex

Commonly occurs when dilating the cervix or when passing the hysteroscope. The prevalence of vagal reaction depends on the ability of the hysteroscopist and on the diameter of the scope. The patient experiences a brief loss of consciousness, preceded by a sense of anticipation. First, there is a period of sympathetic tone, with increased pulse and blood pressure, in anticipation of the stress. Following this, there is a precipitous drop in sympathetic tone, pulse and blood pressure, causing the patient to lose consciousness. Transient bradycardia and few clonic limb jerks may accompany vaso-vagal syncope, but there are usually no sustained injuries. Ordinarily, the patient spontaneously revives after spending a few minutes supine. After full recovery, explain to the patient that this is a common physiological reaction and will have no sequelae. It can be prevented with the administration of 0.6 ml of atropine 20 minutes prior to

commencing the procedure. Atropine is fully effective in completely abolishing the bradycardia and inhibiting vaso-vagal responses. Atropine should not be given if the patient suffers from cardiocirculatory problems.

Cervical trauma

It is best to avoid over dilating the cervix since leakage of the distending media through the cervix and around the hysteroscope then occurs and poor distension makes observation and operating more difficult because of a poor view. Such dilatation is often difficult in nulliparous women with a stenotic cervix. Avoiding cervical dilatation should prove advantageous in reducing the risk of cervical laceration and uterine perforation. However, operative hysteroscopy may need cervical dilatation. Some cervical canals are difficult to negotiate with dilators. Different dilators have a variable amount of curvature to choose from. Some ambulatory procedures may be performed under paracervical block and analgesia.

It is important to remember that diagnostic hysteroscopy performed in the outpatient setting rarely needs cervical dilatation. Also one advantage of the bipolar electrode system is that cervical dilatation is not required. Most diagnostic procedures are performed without analgesia or anaesthesia – even operative ambulatory procedures – especially with the Versascope and especially if one uses the vaginoscopic technique of Bettocchi and Farrugia (see Chapter 3). Cervical trauma is more frequently encountered during a rapid or a difficult dilatation of a stenotic cervix. It is then possible for a tremendous amount of distending media to become intravasated through these rents and into the large vessels of the lower uterine region if they are transected (Table 8.3).

Uterine perforation

Uterine perforation is a rare event. A recent UK Royal College of Obstetricians and Gynaecologists' guideline of taking consent for diagnostic

Table 8.3. Avoidance of cervical trauma

- Do not insert dilators beyond the internal os. The normal cervical canal length to the internal os is 4–5 cm
- Rough cervical dilatation will result in bleeding and endometrial damage

hysteroscopy under general anaesthetic quoted a figure as low as 8/1000 for uterine perforation. For ambulatory procedures, the figure is much lower. In a large systematic review of studies of over 25,000 women, only 4 cases (1/6000) of uterine perforation occurred. Even for inpatient operative procedures, the incidence is low. In the British Mistletoe study, perforation occurred in 6/1000 and 6/1000 of cases, respectively, with roller ball and laser but in 13/1000 and 25/1000 of cases when roller ball and loop or loop alone were used.

The uterus may be perforated by a dilator, the hysteroscope, or an energy source. Management will depend on the size, site of the perforation, and whether there is risk of injury to another organ. Perforation occurs more frequently at the level of the fundus without significant bleeding and should be suspected if the dilator passes to a depth greater than the length of the uterine cavity. Perforation with the hysteroscope should be avoided by always introducing the telescope under direct vision. Simple perforation rarely causes any further damage and may be treated conservatively by admission, observation and appropriate broad-spectrum antibiotics. Laparoscopy may be considered to exclude bleeding. Complex perforation may be made with mechanical or electrical instruments and, therefore, may be associated with injury to adjacent structures including bowel or large vessels. However, energy sources used in the outpatient setting are usually bipolar energy or heat (Thermachoice), which offer reduction of energy spread through the tissue during the procedure. If perforation is suspected,

the energy source should be switched off and the hysteroscope left *in situ* while preparing for laparoscopy. Laparoscopic examination to exclude bowel injury may be all that is necessary. However, in the majority of cases of electrical injury and in all cases where laser has been used, laparotomy and detailed examination of the bowel, pelvic blood vessels and aorta is mandatory.

Haemorrhage

Intra- or postoperative bleeding can be caused by: (i) the tenaculum; (ii) uterine perforation; and (iii) the procedure. Management will depend on the site, severity and cause of the bleeding. Intra-uterine bleeding occurring during the procedure should be immediately obvious and can usually be controlled by spot electrocoagulation (Fig. 8.1).

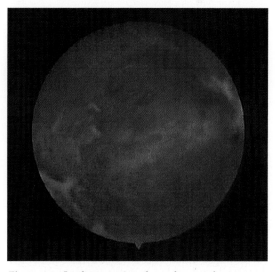

Figure 8.1 Inadequate view due to haemorrhage

If coagulation fails to control the bleeding, the procedure may have to be abandoned and tamponade performed by inserting a Foley catheter and distending the balloon. The catheter should be left *in situ* for a few hours after which the bleeding nearly always stops.

In a large observational clinical study from Italy, 501 women were treated for benign intra-uterine pathologies using an outpatient hystero-scopic procedure, without analgesia or anaesthe-sia. A 5-Fr bipolar electrical electrode was used to treat endometrial polyps ranging between 0.5–4.5 cm, as well as submucosal and partially intramural myomas between 0.6–2.0 cm. No fail-ures or major complications (*i.e.* severe pain, vagal reflex, intravasation, uterine perforation, bleeding) occurred during the procedures.

Less significant bleeding may be caused by tearing of the cervix with the tenaculum or uterine perforation. Lateral tears of the cervix may pro-duce significant bleeding.

Delayed complications of ambulatory hysteroscopy

Infection

An incidence of 2/1000 of infection has been reported in over 4000 diagnostic hysteroscopies. Acute pelvic inflammatory disease is rare following hysteroscopic surgery. The diagnosis is made by the presentation of the classic symptoms and signs and treatment should be by appropriate antibiotics following culture of vaginal swabs and blood (both aerobic and anaerobic).

Vaginal discharge

This is common after any ablative procedure and can sometimes be prolonged (2–3 weeks); however, it is usually self-limiting. Patients should alert their healthcare provider if the vaginal discharges become offensive or if she develops pyrexia, heavy bleeding or severe lower abdominal pain.

Adhesion formation

Intra-uterine adhesions are common especially after myomectomy when two fibroids are situated on opposing uterine walls. In this case, the myomectomy is better performed in stages to prevent adhesion formation. An intra-uterine device and 2 months' administration of oestrogen and progestogen therapy (in the form of combined oral contraceptives) may also help prevent adhesion formation following resection, adhesio-lysis or division of a septum (Fig. 6.5a–f).

FAILURE OF RESOLUTION OF THE PRESENTING SYMPTOMS

The procedure may fail to cure the presenting symptoms. This may be because of poor patient selection or failure of the surgery. Approximately 15% of patients have an early pregnancy loss following septum resection. There is also greater risk of third stage complications. Submucous myomectomy for menorrhagia or infertility gives disappointing results. About 20% of patients have no immediate improvement. Endometrial ablation produces amenorrhoea in about 30% of cases and satisfactory improvement in a further 50%. About 10% will require further surgery, which may be a repeat ablation or hysterectomy. Adhesiolysis for Asherman's syndrome is only curative in about 30–40% of cases. These figures refer to inpatient operative hysteroscopy. There are little outcome data for outpatient operative procedures.

FAILURE TO MAKE AN ACCURATE DIAGNOSIS

This is discussed in Chapter 4.

AVOIDANCE OF COMPLICATIONS

Pre-operative factors to consider

- complexity of procedure

- size of uterus
- the role of Misoprostol when expecting a difficult dilatation
- overall health status and co-morbidity.

Pre-operative optional imaging studies

These may play a role as a diagnostic aid and provide additional information about the cavity that can be useful during surgery.

- hysterosalpingogram
- sonohysterogram

- transvaginal ultrasound
- computerised tomography or magnetic resonance imaging.

Operator's experience

With improved training, experience, and technology, most of these complications can be minimised. There will always be some unavoidable complications as well as difficulties resulting from inexperience. A goal for the future is to teach health professionals how to recognise and treat these complications to ensure the best patient outcome possible.

Key points

➢ The complications of ambulatory hysteroscopy are rare and are seldom life-threatening.

➢ Positioning problems include: damage to soft tissues, nerve injury and deep vein thrombosis.

➢ Uterine perforation is rare but the possibility must be remembered.

➢ To minimise the risk of perforation, bleeding and endometrial damage, do not insert dilators beyond the internal os.

➢ Complications produced by the distension media tend to be specific to hysteroscopic surgery usually under general anaesthesia.

➢ Acute pelvic inflammatory disease is rare following hysteroscopic surgery. However, vaginal discharge is common after any ablative procedure and can sometimes be prolonged (2–3 weeks).

➢ Failure to reach a diagnosis is something that patients should be made aware of pre-procedure.

MULTIPLE CHOICE QUESTIONS

1. **Ambulatory hysteroscopy:**

    Is generally a safe procedure   True/False

    In diagnostic procedures, most complications are rare and seldom
    life-threatening   True/False

| Complications of ambulatory operative procedures are mainly due to fluid intravasation | True/False |
| Operator's experience is irrelevant to complications | True/False |

2. Complications of operative hysteroscopy:

Are related to the type of procedure	True/False
False passage is the most common complication	True/False
Hysteroscopic polypectomy and resection of fibroids are associated with high rates of complications	True/False
Resection of uterine septa has significantly higher complication rate than polypectomy	True/False

3. Complications of excessive absorption of distension media:

With hysteroscopic procedures, occur equally in ambulatory and inpatient settings	True/False
Should be extremely rare if the correct insufflator (hysteroflator) is used	True/False
Cardiac arrhythmias do not occur with diagnostic hysteroscopy using CO_2	True/False
Gas embolism during hysteroscopy is rare but fatal	True/False

4. Fluids as distension media:

Electrolytic solutions (normal saline or lactated Ringer's) can be used in conjunction with monopolar electrosurgical devices	True/False
Electrolytic solutions (normal saline or lactated Ringer's) can be used in conjunction with laser or bipolar energy	True/False
Glycine is used in conjunction with monopolar electrosurgical energy	True/False
Complications of dextran include coagulation disorders	True/False

5. Prevention of fluid extravasation can be accomplished by:

Using appropriate distension media and delivery systems	True/False
Keeping operating times to a minimum	True/False
Keeping fluid pressures as low as possible	True/False
Meticulous fluid balance. The procedure must be abandoned if the deficit rises to 2000 ml	True/False

6. Uterine perforation:

In the British Mistletoe study, perforation occurred in 6/100 cases	True/False
Uterine perforation in ambulatory hysteroscopy is a rare event	True/False
Should be avoided by always introducing the telescope under direct vision	True/False
Laparoscopy should always be performed to exclude bleeding	True/False

7.   Delayed complications of ambulatory hysteroscopy:

Infection, vaginal discharge, adhesion formation and haemorrhage are all
delayed complications of ambulatory hysteroscopy   True/False

Acute pelvic inflammatory disease is rare following hysteroscopic surgery   True/False

Vaginal discharge is common after any ablative procedure   True/False

Vaginal discharge can sometimes be prolonged (2–3 months)   True/False

9 Accuracy of diagnostic ambulatory hysteroscopy

OBJECTIVE: To provide an assessment of the value of hysteroscopy for diagnosis of malignant, premalignant, and benign conditions, relative to ultrasound and endometrial biopsy.

CONTENTS

How test accuracy is assessed
Accuracy of diagnostic hysteroscopy
Comparison with ultrasound scan and
endometrial biopsy

Test combinations
Key points
OSCEs

The main aim of investigations for abnormal uterine bleeding is to exclude endometrial carcinoma and its precursor, endometrial hyperplasia, either complex or atypical. This is because endometrial cancer is associated with abnormal uterine bleeding in over 90% of cases. In addition, identification of benign pathology like polyps and fibroids are also important (Table 9.1). Traditionally, abnormal uterine bleeding had been investigated with dilatation and curettage but, as emphasised throughout this book, there is a trend towards minimally invasive investigations including outpatient hysteroscopy, ultrasound scan and endometrial biopsy. There is a large body of research underpinning these technologies, often with conflicting results. The best way of evaluating endometrial abnormalities remains a subject of a continuing debate. A combination of ultrasound imaging, endoscopy and tissue sampling remain in common use. The authors actively contributed to the existing evidence on the topic and have critically appraised the available literature.

Hysteroscopy provides direct endometrial visualisation of intra-uterine pathology. With improvements in the quality of hysteroscopic technology, a high degree of diagnostic accuracy is being assumed. This chapter provides facts about the real value of hysteroscopic diagnosis.

HOW TEST ACCURACY IS ASSESSED

In studies of test accuracy, the information from the test (hysteroscopy) is compared with a reference standard. The reference standard is the best available method for verifying the presence or absence of the diagnosis, which, in this instance, is histological examination. As shown in Figure 9.1, the term accuracy refers to the amount of agreement between the information from the test under evaluation and the reference standard.

Table 9.1. Differential diagnosis in postmenopausal bleeding

Endometrial pathology
- Endometrial cancer
- Hyperplasia can be simple, complex, or atypical
- Polyps
- Fibroids

Atrophic endometrium – most common diagnosis

Hormonal effect – proliferative or secretory endometrium particularly in hormone replacement
    therapy/tamoxifen users

Cervical, vaginal or vulval pathology

Extra-genital tract source, per rectal bleeding or haematuria

---

Test accuracy can be expressed as sensitivity and specificity, likelihood ratios LRs, diagnostic odds ratio, the area under a receiver operating characteristic curve (ROC curve). See Table 9.2 for definitions and Figure 9.1 for mathematical computation. There is a debate about which measures are preferable and how best to pool them across several studies in a meta-analysis. No single approach is entirely satisfactory. Many experts consider pooling of predictive values, sensitivity and specificity inappropriate, as they do not behave independently. Without going into a long discussion about the pros and cons of various approaches, LRs provides several advantages over other measures when a single threshold for abnormality is used in all studies. For a negative test result, LR < 0.1 is regarded as definitely useful, 0.1–0.2 is regarded as moderately useful, 0.2–0.5 is regarded as slightly useful, and 0.5–1 is regarded as not at all useful. For a positive test result, LR > 10 is regarded as definitely useful, LR 5–10 is regarded as moderately useful, LR 2–5 is regarded as slightly useful, and LR 1–2 is regarded as not at all useful.

The generation of LRs and post-test probabilities represents a more powerful method of establishing the utility of a test. Likelihood ratios are more clinically meaningful because, when they are used in conjunction with information on disease prevalence (pretest probability), they help to generate post-test probabilities as shown in Figures 9.2 and 9.3. A rigorous evaluation of test accuracy studies could help limit healthcare costs by preventing unnecessary testing and by reducing the number of unwanted clinical consequences related to false test results.

ACCURACY OF DIAGNOSTIC HYSTEROSCOPY

When the uterine cavity is adequately visualised, hysteroscopy is highly accurate and thereby clinically useful in the diagnosis of endometrial cancer. The diagnostic accuracy of hysteroscopy for endometrial cancer is such that the LRs are 62 and 0.15 for positive and negative results, respectively. The pretest probability increases, as shown in Figure 9.2, with a positive result and decreases with a negative result as shown in Figure 9.3.

The diagnostic accuracy of hysteroscopy in endometrial cancer and hyperplasia is more modest so that it cannot be included or excluded

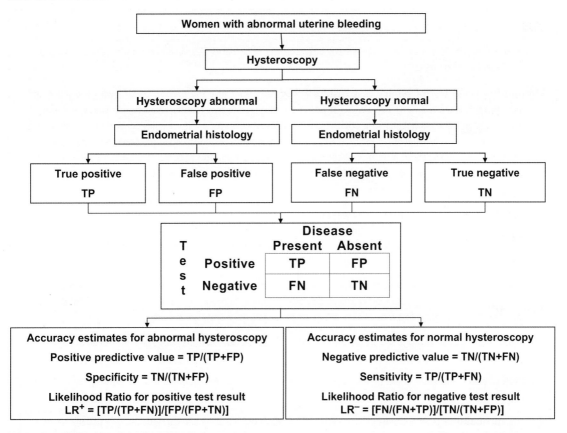

Figure 9.1 Study design for estimation of accuracy of hysteroscopy.

with a high level of certainty. For endometrial cancer and hyperplasia, the pooled LRs are 10 and 0.24 for positive and negative hysteroscopy results, respectively. The probability changes are not as profound with these likelihood ratio values. This relatively inferior performance of hysteroscopy in detecting endometrial disease in comparison to its performance in detecting endometrial cancer is probably because features of hyperplasia are not clearly distinct. For diagnosis of benign submucous fibroids and endometrial polyps, hysteroscopy has quite a high degree of accuracy as shown in Figure 9.4.

Performance of hysteroscopy as a test does not appear to be altered by menopausal status. Compared to the inpatient setting, outpatient hysteroscopy has a marginally higher failure rate, but it appears to have a trend towards improved diagnostic performance. There is a tendency toward improved diagnostic accuracy outpatient hysteroscopy for both endometrial cancer and disease compared with inpatient procedures.

COMPARISON WITH ULTRASOUND AND ENDOMETRIAL BIOPSY

Outpatient, office-based evaluation with endometrial biopsy, transvaginal ultrasonography, saline infusion sonography, and hysteroscopy have supplanted traditional blind dilation and curettage for initial evaluation. A comparison of accuracy of these tests is provided in Figure 9.4. Although endometrial biopsy is accurate and a relatively inexpensive test for identifying endometrial

Table 9.2 Definitions

Accuracy refers to the amount of agreement between the information from the test under evaluation and the reference standard.

Computing accuracy for binary test results: Predictive values give the probability of having a disease and not having a disease among subjects with positive and negative test results, respectively. Sensitivity and specificity give the probability of a positive and a negative test result among subjects with and without disease respectively. Likelihood ratios (LRs) describe the relative probabilities of obtaining a test result in subjects with and without a disease. With several studies to compute accuracy for, and to estimate uncertainty of, the accuracy (its confidence intervals), manual calculations can become tedious. We would suggest using statistical software.

Liklihood ratio (LR) is the ratio of the probability of a positive (or negative) test result in subjects with a disease to the probability of the same test result in subjects without the disease. The LR indicates by how much a given hysteroscopy finding raises or lowers the probability of having endometrial cancer or disease.

Measures of test accuracy are statistics for summarising the accuracy of a test. For binary tests, there are commonly used pairs of accuracy measures: positive and negative predictive values; sensitivity and specificity; and likelihood ratios. Unlike measures of effect, single measures of accuracy are infrequently used.

Negative predictive value is the probability of not having a disease among subjects with negative test results.

Positive predictive value is the probability of having a disease and not having a disease among subjects with positive test results.

Pretest probability is an estimate of probability of disease before tests are carried out. It is usually based on disease prevalence.

Post-test probability is an estimate of probability of disease in the light of information obtained from testing. With accurate tests, the post-test estimates of probabilities change substantially from pretest estimates.

Receiver operating characteristic (ROC) curve is generated by plotting the estimates of sensitivity (true positive rates) against specificity (false positive rates) to characterise the performance of the test. This is a commonly used approach in both primary and secondary research for evaluating diagnostic accuracy of tests. ROC curves can be readily generated from logistic regression modelling and this type of approach has been used in tests with multiple co-variates. The area under the curve (ROC area) determines the accuracy with which the test diagnoses the condition of interest. A ROC area greater than 0.5 suggests some degree of test accuracy, with higher accuracy suggested by an ROC area closer to 1.0 (representing perfect test accuracy).

Reference standard is the best available method for verifying the presence or absence of the diagnosis, which is histological examination in this instance.

Sensitivity gives the probability of a positive test result among subjects with disease.

Specificity gives the probability of a negative test result among subjects without disease.

Systematic review is a research article that identifies relevant studies, appraises their quality and summarises their results using a scientific methodology.

(a) Generating post-test probabilities for a positive test

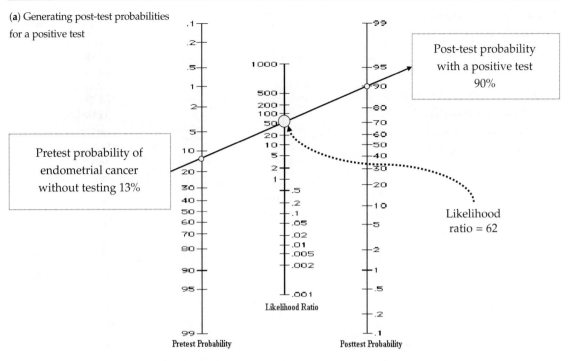

Pretest probability of endometrial cancer without testing 13%

Post-test probability with a positive test 90%

Likelihood ratio = 62

Pretest Probability

Likelihood Ratio

Posttest Probability

Nomogram adapted from N Engl J Med 1975;293:257.

(b) Post-test probabilities of endometrial cancer according to risk groups based on age

Age group	Pretest probability*	Post-test probability[+]
< 50 years	0.5%	24%
51–60 years	1.0%	39%
> 60 years	13.0%	90%

*Obtained from population-based data.

[+]Computed using the formula:

$$\text{Post-test probability} = \frac{\text{Likelihood ratio} \times \text{Pretest probability}}{[1 - \text{Pretest probability} \times (1 - \text{Likelihood ratio})]}$$

Figure 9.2 Change from pretest to post-test probabilities using likelihood ratios. The impact of abnormal hysteroscopy findings (positive hysteroscopy) on the likelihood of endometrial cancer among postmenopausal women with vaginal bleeding. [*Reproduced with permission from*: KS Khan, R Kunz, J Kleijnen, G Antes. *Systematic Reviews to Support Evidence-Based Medicine: How to Review and Apply Findings of Healthcare Research.* London: RSM Press, 2003]

malignancy and premalignancy, it is a poor test for diagnosing benign endometrial abnormalities such as atrophy, polyps, and submucosal fibroids, which are far more common causes of bleeding.

Transvaginal ultrasonography techniques have better accuracy in the identification of benign conditions compared to endometrial biopsy. In comparison, hysteroscopy allows for examination

(a) Generating post-test probabilities
for a negative test

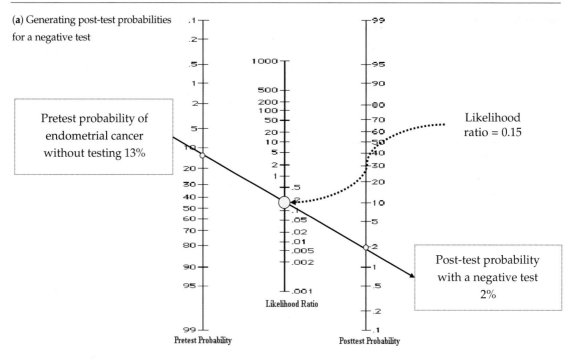

Nomogram adapted from N Engl J Med 1975;293:257.

(b) Post-test probabilities of endometrial cancer according to risk groups based on age

Age group	Pretest probability*	Post-test probability+
< 50 years	0.5%	0%
51–60 years	1.0%	0%
> 60 years	13.0%	2%

*Obtained from population-based data.

+Computed using the formula:

$$\text{Post-test probability} = \frac{\text{Likelihood ratio x Pretest probability}}{[1 - \text{Pretest probability x } (1 - \text{Likelihood ratio})]}$$

Figure 9.3 The impact of normal hysteroscopy findings (negative hysteroscopy) on the likelihood of endometrial cancer among postmenopausal women with vaginal bleeding. [*Reproduced with permission from*: KS Khan, R Kunz, J Kleijnen, G Antes. *Systematic Reviews to Support Evidence-Based Medicine: How to Review and Apply Findings of Healthcare Research*. London: RSM Press, 2003]

of the whole endometrial cavity, lower segment and cervical canal. Hysteroscopy can detect small polyp or submucous fibroids, which have been missed by endometrial biopsy, or blind curettage. Hysteroscopy is considered the gold standard for the accurate detection of these intra-uterine pathologies for its superiority in directly visualising these lesions.

Ultrasound scan, particularly the transvaginal route, is frequently used to assess endometrial

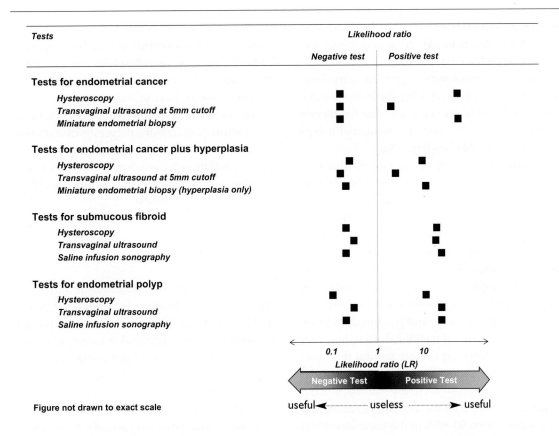

Figure 9.4 Comparison of accuracy of hysteroscopy with other modalities for diagnosis of malignant, premalignant and benign condition among women with abnormal uterine bleeding. The LR indicated by how much a given diagnostic test finding will raise or lower the probability of having the disease. The vertical line drawn at LR value of 1.0 represent 'no effect'. With a positive test, an LR >1 increases the probability that the disease is present. The greater the LR, the larger the increase in the probability of the disease and the more clinically useful the test result. With a negative hysteroscopy, an LR <1 decreases the probability that the disease is present. The smaller the LR, the larger the decrease and the more clinically useful the test result.

thickness, endometrial and myometrial consistency and abnormalities of endometrial morphology like submucosal fibroids or polyps, *etc*. Transvaginal ultrasonography has better quality of image because of its higher frequency, which allows greater image resolution at the expense of decreased depth of penetration. The average endometrial thickness for normal postmenopausal women tends to be < 4 mm, those with endometrial polyp of 10 mm, those with endometrial hyperplasia of 14 mm and endometrial carcinoma of 20 mm. Using a 5-mm threshold to define abnormal endometrial thickening, generally it can be concluded that transvaginal ultrasound can accurately identify postmenopausal women with vaginal bleeding who are highly unlikely to have significant endometrial disease so that endometrial sampling or even hysteroscopy may be unnecessary. The prediction of endometrial pathology based on ultrasound scan in premenopausal women is not reliable because of great overlap between the normal range and those with endometrial pathology.

The role of sonohysterography or saline infusion sonography is developing. It involves instillation of 5–15 ml of normal saline into the uterine cavity for better detection of endometrial polyps and submucous fibroids (Fig. 6.2a).

Endometrial biopsy is accurate for diagnosing neoplasia. The main purpose of obtaining an endometrial biopsy or aspirate is to exclude endometrial pathology such as hyperplasia, disordered endometrium or malignancies. Most endometrial biopsies can be performed in outpatient or office clinics and have the advantage of being simple, quick, safe, convenient and avoiding the need for anaesthesia. Furthermore, the device is disposable and is a hundred times less costly than a conventional dilatation and curettage; however, it is more painful than outpatient hysteroscopy. Outpatient endometrial biopsy has modest accuracy in diagnosing endometrial hyperplasia. The sample adequacy rate ranges from 90–95% in the premenopausal group. For postmenopausal patients, the adequacy rate is significantly lower probably because of the atrophic endometrium. Outpatient endometrial sampling has a procedure failure rate as well as a tissue-yield failure rate, each of approximately 10%. It should be noted that yield failures are to be expected in women with atrophic endometrial lining, whereas failure to obtain tissue would be less likely if cancer was present. The false-negative rate for endometrial carcinoma is low so endometrial biopsy is accurate in excluding endometrial carcinoma. In general, additional assessment of the endometrial cavity should be undertaken, especially if symptoms persist or intra-uterine structural abnormalities are suspected.

It has been suggested that routine endometrial biopsy is not necessary at the initial investigation for menorrhagia (heavy, but regular, periods). In all women with abnormal uterine bleeding at or above the age of 40 years the incidence of endometrial cancer and hyperplasia increases sharply. The woman's risk of having endometrial carcinoma should be assessed considering factors other than age. Patients with obesity, polycystic ovarian syndrome, unopposed oestrogen therapy, tamoxifen therapy and those patients with persistent or long-standing abnormal uterine bleeding should be offered endometrial biopsy.

TEST COMBINATIONS

There remains an on-going debate about the choice between ultrasound, endometrial biopsy and hysteroscopy in the management of women presenting with abnormal uterine bleeding. Some have recommended test combinations, for example pelvic ultrasound scan and/or outpatient hysteroscopy. The true clinical value of the added tests lies in the additional information over and above what was already known from the history, examination and prior testing. Ultrasonography is considered less invasive than hysteroscopy and it is accurate in ruling out endometrial cancer and hyperplasia in postmenopausal women. Ambulatory hysteroscopy is accurate in ruling in endometrial cancer and hyperplasia. Thus transvaginal ultrasound scan may be employed as an initial test followed by hysteroscopy in women with abnormal uterine bleeding who have a positive result on ultrasound scanning. Endometrial sampling may also be considered as an initial test for excluding malignancy. Whether sonography or endometrial biopsy is used initially depends on the physician's assessment of patient risk, the nature of the physician's practice, the availability of high-quality sonography, and patient preference.

Key points

➢ Hysteroscopy is highly accurate and, thereby, clinically useful in the diagnosis of endometrial cancer. However, the diagnostic accuracy of hysteroscopy in endometrial hyperplasia is more modest. For polyps and submucous fibroids, hysteroscopy is considered virtually a gold standard.

➢ Performance of hysteroscopy as a test does not appear to be altered by menopausal status.

➢ Compared to the inpatient setting, outpatient hysteroscopy has a marginally higher failure rate.

➢ There is a tendency toward improved diagnostic accuracy with outpatient hysteroscopy compared to inpatient procedures.

➢ The chance of endometrial carcinoma in women below the age of 40 years is low and endometrial assessment is not warranted unless there are associated risk factors for endometrial carcinoma or if the symptoms are persistent/long-standing or symptoms fail to respond to medical treatment.

➢ The relative roles of ultrasound, endometrial biopsy and hysteroscopy and their combinations for diagnosis of pathology remain a topic of debate, but hysteroscopy is evidently superior in many respects.

OBJECTIVE STRUCTURED CLINICAL EXAMINATIONS (OSCEs)

1. **You are asked to see a patient with 3 months' history of postmenopausal bleeding. Physical examination does not reveal any abnormality. The patient has heard that she may have polyps. Read the following abstract and answer the subsequent questions about this patient.**

ABSTRACT

Study objective: To assess the diagnostic potential of ultrasound in identifying polyps in postmenopausal bleeding.

Design: Prospective evaluation.

Setting: Outpatient ultrasound and hysteroscopy department of a university-affiliated hospital.

Patients: Two hundred women with an endometrial thickness assessment on ultrasound and in menopause for at least 1 year.

Interventions: Transvaginal ultrasound and office hysteroscopy, with eye-directed biopsy specimens obtained with a 5-mm, continuous-flow operative hysteroscope, and performed without anaesthesia. Hysteroscopy served as the 'gold' standard for diagnosis of polyps.

Measurements and main results: Endometrial polyps were seen on hysteroscopy in 35 women. Among 150 women, the endometrium was regular with thickness less than 4 mm. Of these, 15 had endometrial polyps. Among 50 women, the endometrium was irregular and/or thickness was 4 mm or more. Of these, 20 had endometrial polyps.

Conclusion: Hysteroscopy allows a proper diagnosis of endometrial polyps.

Now answer the following questions about this patient.

1 (i) Before performing any investigations, what is the probability that there is an endometrial polyp?
This question is answered by finding out the proportion of women with polyps in the study sample.

     A.   about 1.75%

     B.   about 17.5%

     C.   about 20%

     D.   virtually 100%   *The correct answer is:*

1 (ii) An ultrasound examination has been carried out that shows endometrial thickness of more than 4 mm. What is the probability that there is an endometrial polyp?

     E.   virtually 100%

     F.   about 4%

     G.   about 20%

     H.   about 40%   *The correct answer is:*

1 (iii) A student asks you to show how a 2 x 2 table (shown below) can be generated comparing ultrasound and hysteroscopic diagnosis.

	Hysteroscopy:polyp	Hysteroscopy:no polyp	
Ultrasound positive	True positive (TP)	False positive (FP)	TP+FP
Ultrasound negative	False negative (FN)	True negative (TN)	FN+TN
	TP+FN	FP+TN	Total

Which one of the following 4 tables fits the data presented in the paper?

Table A

	Hysteroscopy:polyp	Hysteroscopy:no polyp	
Ultrasound positive	20	30	50
Ultrasound negative	135	15	150
	155	45	200 patients

Table B

	Hysteroscopy:polyp	Hysteroscopy:no polyp	
Ultrasound positive	20	15	35
Ultrasound negative	30	135	160
	50	150	200 patients

Table C

	Hysteroscopy:polyp	Hysteroscopy:no polyp	
Ultrasound positive	20	30	50
Ultrasound negative	15	135	150
	35	165	200 patients

Table D

	Hysteroscopy:polyp	Hysteroscopy:no polyp	
Ultrasound positive	15	30	45
Ultrasound negative	20	135	155
	35	165	200 patients

The correct table is:

1 (iv) You perform a hysteroscopy. Your view of the entire cavity is satisfactory. You see both tubal ostea clearly. You find normal-looking endometrium without any irregularities. You do not see any polyps. In the light of your findings:

    A.   You must arrange for the patient to have hysteroscopy and curettage under anaesthesia.

    B.   You can re-assure the patient that there are no polyps.

The correct answer is:

2. **You are asked to see a 64-year-old patient with postmenopausal bleeding. Physical examination does not reveal any abnormality. Regarding endometrial cancer, read the attached abstract and answer the following questions about this patient.**

ABSTRACT

Study objectives: The fundamental objective of this study was to determine the true value of hysteroscopy in the assessment of women with postmenopausal bleeding, namely in the diagnosis/exclusion of endometrial carcinoma.

Study methods: 158 women with postmenopausal bleeding were studied with a rigid hysteroscope of 6 mm in external diameter for diagnostic purpose and for biopsy under direct vision. The uterine cavity was distended with CO_2 gas insufflations. Only a paracervical block with lidocaine was used. In all 158 cases, a biopsy was performed and the 'hysteroscopic diagnosis' was compared with the histological diagnosis. True and false positives as well as true and false negatives were calculated and, subsequently, the sensitivity, specificity, negative and positive predictive values, and overall efficiency were all evaluated. Prevalence is also indicated.

Results: The mean age of the women was 64.2 years, with a range of 40–83 years. We found 14 cases of endometrial carcinoma. The prevalence was 8.8%. 14 true positives, 17 false positives, 126 true negatives and 1 false negative were obtained. From the 17 false positives, 4 had a histological diagnosis of simple hyperplasia with cysts, 5 of glandular hyperplasia, and 8 had a normal histology. The false negative had a 'hysteroscopic diagnosis' of endometrial hyperplasia.

Conclusions: Our results show hysteroscopy to be a method with good sensitivity (93.3%), good overall efficiency (88.6%), and an excellent negative predictive value (99.2%). The specificity was 88.1%, and the positive predictive value was 45.1%. Because of the 'hysteroscopic diagnosis' of the false negative, we can conclude that the negative predictive value was virtually 100%.

Now answer the following questions about this patient.

2 (i)   Before performing hysteroscopy, what is the probability that there is endometrial cancer?

     A.   about 8.8%

     B.   about 88.6%

     C.   about 45.1%

     D.   virtually 100%   *The correct answer is:*

2 (ii) A student asks you to show how a 2 x 2 table (shown below) can be generated comparing hysteroscopy and histological diagnosis.

	Histology:cancer	Histology:not cancer	
Hysteroscopy positive	True positive (TP)	False positive (FP)	TP+FP
Hysteroscopy negative	False negative (FN)	True negative (TN)	FN+TN
	TP+FN	FP+TN	Total

Which one of the 4 tables fits the data presented in the paper?

Table A

	Histology:cancer	Histology:not cancer	
Hysteroscopy positive	126	17	143
Hysteroscopy negative	1	14	15
	127	143	158 patients

Table B

	Histology:cancer	Histology:not cancer	
Hysteroscopy positive	1	17	18
Hysteroscopy negative	14	126	140
	15	143	158 patients

Table C

	Histology:cancer	Histology:not cancer	
Hysteroscopy positive	14	17	31
Hysteroscopy negative	1	126	127
	15	143	158 patients

Table D

	Histology:cancer	Histology:not cancer	
Hysteroscopy positive	14	1	15
Hysteroscopy negative	17	126	143
	31	127	158 patients

The correct table is:

2 (iii) You perform a hysteroscopy. Your findings reveal increased endometrial thickness, abnormal vascularisation, and irregularities. You are concerned that the patient might have cancer. In light of your findings, you arrange for the patient to have hysteroscopy and curettage under anaesthesia.

What is the probability that cancer will be present on histology?

A.   17/31

B.   126/127

C.   14/31

D.   1/127   *The correct answer is:*

2 (iv) If the hysteroscopy were negative, what would be the probability of missing a cancer?

A.   17/31

B.   126/127

C.   14/31

D.   1/127   *The correct answer is:*

3. **You are asked to see a patient with postmenopausal bleeding for 3 months. Physical examination does not reveal any abnormality. The patient has heard that she may have cancer of the lining of the womb. Read the attached abstracts, consider the information below, and answer the following questions about this patient.**

ABSTRACT 1

Study of: Transvaginal sonography and progesterone challenge for identifying endometrial pathology in postmenopausal women.

Objective: To evaluate the usefulness of transvaginal sonographic (TVS) measurement of endometrial thickness for identifying endometrial pathology in postmenopausal women.

Methods: 284 postmenopausal women were examined by TVS: 130 asymptomatic women (group A) and 154 with uterine bleeding (group B). Endometrial thickness > 5 mm was considered pathological. All women with abnormal endometrium from group A and all women from group B underwent D&C.

Results: 107 patients from group B had abnormal sonographic and histological findings – benign (hyperplasia, polyp) or malignant (endometrial cancer). There was no cancer in cases with endometrial thickness <= 6 mm. The sensitivity and specificity of TVS for detecting endometrial pathology were 99% and 59%, respectively, if the cut-off limit of 5 mm was used.

Conclusion: TVS is a simple, well-tolerated, safe and reliable method for identifying endometrial pathology in postmenopausal women.

Consider the following information and definitions used in diagnostic studies:

2 x 2 table

	Hysteroscopy or ultrasound		
	Test result positive	Test result negative	
Histology cancer	True positive (TP)	False positive (FP)	TP+FP
Histology benign	False negative (FN)	True negative (TN)	FN+TN
	TP+FN	FP+TN	Total

Sensitivity

This is the proportion of those people who really have the disease who are correctly identified as such (TP/TP+FN). For 'sensitivity' to be 100% there must be no false-negative cases. Thus a negative 'sensitivity' test rules out disease.

Specificity

This is the proportion of those subjects who really do not have disease who are correctly identified as such (TN/TN+FP). For 'specificity' to be 100% there must be no false-positive cases. A positive 'specificity' test rules in disease.

3 (i) You have a recent study (Abstract 1) about the accuracy of ultrasound at a 5-mm threshold for abnormality for the detection of endometrial cancer. What are the reported values for:

    (A)   Sensitivity   ---------------------------------------

    (B)   Specificity   ---------------------------------------

3 (ii) You have another recent study (Abstract 2) about the accuracy of hysteroscopy for the detection of endometrial cancer.

ABSTRACT 2

Study of: Hysteroscopic evaluation of menopausal patients with sonographic assessment of endometrium.

Aim: To evaluate and compare the diagnostic precision of hysteroscopy in a group of menopausal women in whom D&C was performed.

Methods: A Hamou type II CO_2 hysteroscope was used to evaluate the endocervical canal and the uterine cavity, followed by endometrial sampling.

Results: 39 women were assessed using hysteroscopy and endometrial biopsy. Histopathology results were available for diagnosis in 29 of them (74.3%). In the remaining 10 patients, the hysteroscopic diagnosis was atrophic endometrium. The sensitivity and specificity for hysteroscopy were 53.7% and 96.9%, respectively.

Conclusions: These significant results indicate that this simplified endoscopic method surpasses all blind hospital or office endometrial sampling methods. Therefore, we suggest that hysteroscopy should be the initial assessment tool for any type of indication requiring endometrial and uterine cavity assessment.

What are the reported values for:

    (a)   Sensitivity   -----------------------------------

    (b)   Specificity   -----------------------------------

3 (iii) Considering the above information, what do you think about the relative diagnostic value of the two tests?

    (a)   Ultrasound is very suitable for the exclusion (ruling out) of the disease under question (endometrial cancer).

    (b)   With ultrasound, the probability that the disease under question (*i.e.* cancer) is present despite a negative test result is very low.

    (c)   Hysteroscopy is very suitable for the exclusion (ruling out) of the disease under question (endometrial cancer).

    (d)   With hysteroscopy, the probability that the disease under question (*i.e.* cancer) is present despite a negative test result is very low.

    A.   All statements (a–d) are incorrect.

    B.   The first statement (a) is correct, the second, third and fourth statements (b–d) are incorrect.

    C.   The second and third statement (b,c) are correct, the first and fourth statement (a,d) are incorrect.

    D.   The first and second statements (a,b) are correct, the third and forth statements (c,d) are incorrect.

    E.   All statements (a–d) are correct.   *The correct answer is:*

10 Risk management for ambulatory hysteroscopy

OBJECTIVE: To provide an overview of patient safety issues in an ambulatory hysteroscopy service.

CONTENTS
Patient safety culture
Background to risk management theory

Risk management in ambulatory hysteroscopy
Key points

PATIENT SAFETY CULTURE

As hysteroscopy has dramatically advanced over the last decade shifting the focus in healthcare away from inpatient diagnosis and treatment, the implementation of risk management and clinical governance processes has also escalated with a view to increasing patient safety. The inclusion of all ambulatory services within this safety framework is important, even though ambulatory hysteroscopy is generally considered low-risk. This chapter will give an overview of the risk management theories that underpin current risk management strategy and their application to hysteroscopy services.

Patient safety is at the very core of risk management. It is the first and foremost domain of healthcare. Hysteroscopists would not dispute this stance, as they do not wish their patients to be harmed during the course of their care. However, research has shown that patients are harmed all too frequently with up to 11% of them experiencing an adverse event whilst in hospital. Of these, up to 50% of the incidents are preventable.

When performing ambulatory hysteroscopy patient safety objectives should be undertaken for all of the following component tasks:

- Appropriate patient selection and clinic booking

- Adequate preparation of the patient for the procedure

- Undertake hysteroscopic procedure(s) successfully

- An accurate diagnosis and appropriate treatment

- Avoid procedure-related harm to the patient (and staff)

- Effective communication of results to patient and carers

- Plan and communicate further management.

When the procedure is broken down in this way, it is clear that errors or mistakes can happen at any stage. For an ambulatory hysteroscopy service to achieve the above objectives, it cannot operate in isolation from other areas of health provision, for example clinic administration, gynaecological pathology, primary care, *etc.* Interfaces between these areas represent potential barriers to patient safety.

Risk management involves identifying risk, measuring or quantifying it, and then either to eliminate it or to ameliorate it in some way. Identifying risks can rely on historical data, for example from incident reporting, or previous problems experienced either in the same clinic or elsewhere. This, in turn, relies on incidents being reported as well as information systems and networks being in place. For example, an incident happening in a different part of the hospital, remote from hysteroscopy, may have implications for it; however, if the risk management infrastructure is not in place to communicate those risks, no lessons will be learnt.

BACKGROUND TO RISK MANAGEMENT THEORY

Outside healthcare, other industries, such as aviation, have been active in risk management for years. Most theories and academic logic underpinning risk management have resulted from close studies of adverse events occurring in these industries. Risk management in healthcare can learn from the wealth of parallel experience from other sectors. It is clear that, when an adverse incident occurs, it is no good just looking at the immediate event that preceded the incident to understand its cause, as there are multiple underlying factors that may have 'allowed' the accident to happen (Fig. 10.1).

With advances in technology, errors are more likely to be 'human'. Psychologists divide human error into two causally determined groups. First, 'execution failures' due to slips and lapses, where an action deviates from the current intention, often due to attentional problems. The second group is that due to mistakes (*i.e.* planning or problem-solving failures) which can be either rule-based mistakes (*e.g.* the misapplication of a good rule) or knowledge-based mistakes. Improving the quality and delivery of information in the workplace may reduce errors. Distinct from errors are deliberate violations, which are intended deviations from safe practices and may occur in order to cut corners or because

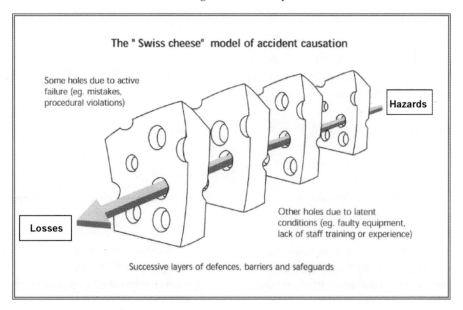

Figure 10.1 Reason's model of accident causation.

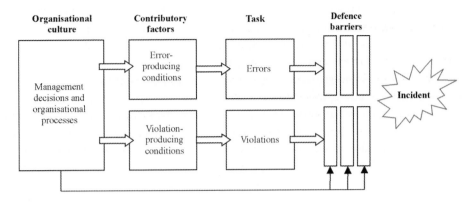

Figure 10.2 Stages of development of an organisational accident.

the usual course of action seems inappropriate to a particular situation. Violations may require organisational and motivational remedies as shown in Table 10.1.

Finally there are active and latent failures. An active failure will have an immediate consequence (*e.g.* giving the wrong medication); these are the errors and violations committed by those on the shop floor in direct contact with patients.

A latent failure may be created as a result of a wrong decision taken at a high level within an organisation some time earlier, only becoming

apparent in a particular set of circumstances which breach the systems defences.

Figure 10.2 shows the anatomy of an incident. The accident sequence starts on the left with organisational latent failures, which when transmitted to the workplace help to create the conditions in which errors and violations thrive (*e.g.* understaffing, high work-load). If these errors/violations then penetrate the defences, an incident can occur.

This model provides an understanding of the aetiology of an incident. This approach concen-

Table 10.1 Examples of learning from errors to minimise risk

Case 1
A patient undergoing a hysteroscopy complained of feeling unwell. The trainee hysteroscopist continued with the procedure, considering that the examination would be finished very soon. The patient became faint, had a major vaso-vagal collapse and went on to fit. She received supportive therapy and subsequently made a full recovery. A guideline was introduced, which states that when a patient complains of feeling unwell, immediately stop performing the examination, move the patient's couch to the head-down position and administer oxygen and atropine if required.

Case 2
A hysteroscope was introduced into the patient's uterus and an instrument advanced down the operating channel, situated at 12-o'clock on the hysteroscope. A significant perforation of the anterior uterine wall occurred. Training is now given to direct the hysteroscope posteriorly within the uterus to allow room to visualise the safe passage of an instrument out of the anterior channel.

trates on the conditions under which individuals work (such as organisational factors, team factors, task factors, situational and individual factors) and builds up defences to avert errors or to mitigate their effects. This model underpins a variety of risk management tools including 'root cause analysis' for the investigation of serious adverse healthcare incidents and 'near misses'. Such analyses enable us to learn important lessons about the prevention of future incidents and harm to patients. They have demonstrated that the following conditions are particularly likely to be associated with errors:

- Unfamiliarity with the task
- Shortage of time
- Poor human/equipment interface
- Inexperience
- Poor procedures
- Inadequate checking.

RISK MANAGEMENT IN AMBULATORY HYSTEROSCOPY

For an ambulatory hysteroscopy service, a regular risk assessment will enable the identification of risks. Whilst historical data from incident reporting are very useful, a more pro-active approach is essential if 'hidden' or obscure risks are to be identified. A framework for performing risk assessment may involve mapping a 'patient's journey' through the hysteroscopy service, assessing the following areas for clinical and non-clinical risks:

- Environment, *e.g.* equipment, medicine use, infection control
- Staffing, *e.g.* number, training
- Patient assessment, *e.g.* availability of medical records, documentation
- Patient treatment, *e.g.* guidelines and consent
- Discharge/follow-up arrangements.

Each of the assessment criteria should be referenced where possible to good practice

guidelines. Specific areas for risk management in ambulatory hysteroscopy are covered below.

Patient selection

Sticking to the rules regarding patient selection can optimise patient safety as well as reducing delays due to wasted appointments. Thorough history taking may identify those at higher risk of pelvic infection in whom swab results should be obtained first. If there is any possibility of pregnancy, a pregnancy test needs to be performed. The referring clinician must perform a speculum examination to ensure that it is easy to visualise the cervix and that it is normal. We have found cervical carcinomas at the time of hysteroscopy where this assessment before referral has clearly not been adequate.

Documentation

A thorough review of a patient's history and a pelvic examination are fundamental requirements for effective service provision. Whilst different approaches exist, the unit in Bradford pioneered GP direct access to hysteroscopic outpatient services. Primary care colleagues, who commence the assessment and consent process, document their findings and the patient's history, and the patient brings her own booklet containing her details to her appointment. This booklet is also used to document the hysteroscopic and examination findings, thus providing a complete record of the episode of care.

The booklet can then be retained within the hospital record, and a summary letter of the episode and findings sent to the referring practitioner. Pathways for the effective communication of outstanding results also need to be developed.

The hysteroscopy booklet can also be adapted for use as a care pathway, which helps to ensure that care given is uniform and of high quality and that important pre-procedure screens for infection and possible pregnancy are not overlooked.

Consent

Consent is best viewed as a process that commences at the decision to investigate the patient further by hysteroscopy. Good evidence is now available to demonstrate the acceptability of outpatient versus inpatient hysteroscopy, when assessed by patient satisfaction. This study also demonstrated that a patient's recovery was quicker after an outpatient hysteroscopy and these issues should be highlighted to patients when discussing choices with them.

The UK Royal College of Obstetricians and Gynaecologists (RCOG) have produced guidance on obtaining valid consent, which ideally should be taken by a practitioner capable of performing the procedure. In addition, a new RCOG guideline will be produced relating to consent for diagnostic hysteroscopy in the outpatient setting. This follows the structure of the UK Department of Health consent form and could be produced as a procedure-specific consent form for inclusion in a hysteroscopic care pathway booklet (see Chapter 4).

Training

Guidance and established schedules for training doctors and nurses to perform hysteroscopy exist and are discussed elsewhere. Training for medical equipment use is also imperative in all settings. A lack of familiarity with the equipment is a factor associated with adverse clinical outcomes. Besides putting patients at high risk for injury, clinicians who use a device they are not familiar with are placing themselves in legal jeopardy. A 45-year-old patient undergoing a diagnostic hysteroscopy in the US died from massive air embolism after incorrect connection of the gas flow apparatus resulting from lack of training. Practitioners should also undertake annual training drills for the rare, unforeseen emergencies, which may arise such as collapse, anaphylaxis and haemorrhage.

New procedures

Healthcare professionals are responsible for notifying the UK National Institute for Clinical Excellence (NICE) when considering use of a procedure that they have not used before, and for applying any guidance on existing procedures to meet the needs of individual patients.

If the procedure has already been notified to NICE, then the clinician should follow any guidance given. The only exception to this is when the procedure is being used only within a protocol approved by a Research Ethics Committee (REC). In this case, notification is not required, as patients are protected by the REC's scrutiny. As there may be a considerable period between the notification of a procedure and the issuing of Interventional Procedures Guidance, NICE produces guidance as precautions a clinician should employ in such circumstances.

Key points

➢ The hysteroscopy service needs to operate within a safety framework and co-ordinate with primary care and allied departments in order to operate effectively.

➢ Identified risks or clinical incidents need to be managed through a robust risk management system to develop safe solutions and prevent future occurrences.

➢ Patient selection, documentation and obtaining consent can have potential pitfalls in safe practice.

➢ Lack of familiarity with equipment is a factor associated with adverse clinical outcomes.

➢ Guidance should be followed regarding the introduction of new clinical procedures.

11 Training in ambulatory hysteroscopy

OBJECTIVE: To provide teachers developing courses with an overview of training programmes for nurses, general practitioners, doctors in training and practising specialists interested in continuing professional development.

Formal hysteroscopy training programmes and accreditation are rapidly expanding among gynaecologists. Trained nurse hysteroscopists and general practitioners are pushing the boundaries even further by performing diagnostic procedures independently and beginning to offer treatments. This chapter provides an overview of various approaches to training in ambulatory hysteroscopy giving training opportunities and guidance to teachers. Training structures vary considerably between countries but the general principles of sound educational courses are universal. The curricula described in this chapter can be easily adapted to meet local training needs. In general, as shown in Table 11.1, a distinction has to be made between two types of training programmes.

1. Diagnostic hysteroscopy training programme: This may be undertaken by any interested professional – a nurse, a general practitioner or a gynaecologist. The training should focus mainly on hysteroscopy as a diagnostic procedure for women with abnormal uterine bleeding.

2. Advanced hysteroscopic surgery training programme: This should be particularly directed at gynaecologists, either in training or qualified specialists, interested in providing treatment for abnormal uterine bleeding. The structured training should be delivered under supervision of a preceptor to inculcate operative skills in an ambulatory setting.

Whatever the training programmes, trainees should progress through a structured educational system with opportunities for increasing responsibility, appropriate supervision, formal instruction, and critical assessment and evaluation.

SPECIALIST NURSE HYSTEROSCOPIST

The role of nurses is expanding world-wide. Nurses are performing tasks that have previously been

Table 11.1. Outcomes of two types of training programme

A **diagnostic hysteroscopy trainee** should be:

- Able to recognise normal and abnormal endometrial appearances

- Able to correlate the findings with the presenting symptoms, endocrine status or pathology

- Competent in ambulatory hysteroscopic techniques

- Aware of diagnostic hysteroscopic complications, their presentations and management

- Able to establish a diagnosis and formulate a plan of action

- Able to communicate effectively information about diagnostic hysteroscopy to patients including discussion on alternate tests

In addition to the above, a **surgical hysteroscopy trainee** should also be:

- Able to undertake hysteroscopic management, where appropriate

- Aware of operative hysteroscopic complications, their prevention and management

- Able to communicate effectively information about hysteroscopic surgery to the patient, including discussion of alternate treatments available

the province of doctors across primary and secondary care and within medical and surgical specialities. It is clear that expanding the role of the nurse is essential to keep the health service afloat.

Within gynaecology, there are nurse practitioners working in the areas of infertility, menopause, and oncology and there are nurses performing colposcopy. In the UK, colposcopy training for doctors became mandatory and structured in 1997. The Royal College of Obstetricians and Gynaecologists (RCOG) and British Society for Colposcopy and Cervical Pathology (BSCCP) offered nurses training programmes and joint accreditation. Nurse colposcopists diagnose and, in some cases, treat benign and pre-malignant lesions of the cervix independently. Similar developments are taking place in ambulatory hysteroscopy.

In 2000, the British Society for Gynaecological Endoscopy (BSGE) in partnership with Bradford University developed a nurse hysteroscopy training programme. This training programme has an exit examination to test knowledge and skills, and attracts academic credit. This programme gives the trainees all the knowledge and skills they will need to advise women regarding their gynaecological symptoms and to perform diagnostic hysteroscopy in outpatient clinics or under general anaesthesia. Each trainee completes over 12–18 months a logbook of cases performed, achieves various competencies and provides case studies of their practice. Passing the programme's assessment allows the trainee to practice independently. This book will prepare trainees for this assessment. Re-accreditation takes place every 3 years.

Table 11.2. Topics covered by the British Society for Gynaecological Endoscopy (BSGE)/Bradford University hysteroscopy course

Premenopausal topics	Postmenopausal topics
• Fibroids	• Postmenopausal bleeding
• Polyps	• Hormone replacement therapy
• Outpatient hysteroscopy	• Menopause
• Pain relief/pelvic pain	• Endometrial cancer
• Endometriosis	• Cervical cancer
• Infertility	**Further topics**
• Resuscitation	• Tamoxifen
• Complications	• Hysterectomy
• Indications/contra-indications	• Presentation skills
• Safety issues	• How to pass an Objective Structured Clinical Examination (OSCE)
• Sterilisation issues	
• Endometrial ablation	
• Medical management of menstrual problems	
• Mirena	

A CURRICULUM FOR TRAINING IN DIAGNOSTIC HYSTEROSCOPY

The course described below is useful for gynaecologists, nurses and general practitioners to gain competence to provide ambulatory hysteroscopy services independently. This programme has trained specialist nurse hysteroscopists and general practitioners. We describe the curriculum of this course in detail below as an example of a programme for training in diagnostic hysteroscopy.

Theoretical training

Theoretical training may be delivered over 10 days in 3 visits spread over a 6-month period as at Bradford. The teaching method should use problem-based learning. This enables the trainees to develop the skills of critical thinking, clinical decision-making and prepares them for independent practice. The trainees also have access to the Internet, CD-ROMs, journals, textbooks and a first-class library. At Bradford, the first visit lasts 5 days and covers pre-menopausal topics. The second visit lasts 3 days and covers postmenopausal topics. The last visit is for 2 days and covers surgery and OSCE training. Table 11.2 shows the topics covered. The syllabus for theoretical modules is shown in Table 11.3.

Practical training

This should be undertaken by the trainee in their own hospital under the supervision of recognised trainers. The trainer should be a member of the BSGE and an experienced hysteroscopist. The

Table 11.3 Theoretical hysteroscopy modules

1. Anatomy and physiology of the normal uterus
2. The abnormal uterus
3. Cervical abnormality
4. Menorrhagia
5. Pelvic pain
6. Infertility
7. Endometrial pre-malignancy and malignancy
8. Evidence-based practice
9. Medicolegal and ethical considerations
10. Menopause and hormone replacement therapy
11. Equipment
12. Histology
13. Analgesia and anaesthesia
14. Miscellaneous

Table 11.4 Practical hysteroscopy modules

1. Preliminary skills
2. Hysteroscopic examination
3. The normal uterus
4. The abnormal uterus
5. Practical procedures
6. Complications
7. Administration
8. Communication skills
9. Audit and clinical governance

trainee is expected to complete a set number of procedures at each level:

- 25 observed cases
- 50–100 cases under direct supervision
- 50–100 cases under indirect supervision.

The progress between stages should be guided by assessments to be undertaken by trainee and trainer together. At the end of each training session during indirect supervision, the trainer should be asked to discuss each case with the trainee to check the diagnosis and treatment advised. It is invaluable to have video recording to aid in this discussion.

There are 9 practical modules (Table 11.4) with 4 levels of competence to achieve (Table 11.5).

Level 1 – observe the practice

Level 2 – perform the task under direct supervision

Level 3 – perform the task under indirect supervision

Level 4 – perform the task independently.

Trainees are advised to hold monthly meetings with their trainers to go through the logbook. The trainers may need to provide additional tuition if required by the trainee.

Exit examination and re-accreditation

The trainee has to produce 10 case studies of 500 words each on a variety of different topics. The logbooks and case studies constitute portfolios of learning achievement for assessment. The exit examination at Bradford takes the form of a 12-station OSCE circuit. The circuit tests the trainees' theoretical and practical knowledge and communication skills. It is both rigorous and robust. On passing this examination, the trainee is awarded a certificate of competence awarded jointly by the BSGE and Bradford University. Following certification, the qualified hysteroscopist must re-accredit in 3 years by completing 100 cases per year, audit practice, attending a BSGE-approved meeting annually, and remaining a member of the BSGE.

Table 11.5. Diagnostic hysteroscopy assessments

SKILL	Competence levels				Preceptor to sign and date when competence achieved
	Level 1 Observed	Level 2 Directly supervised	Level 3 Indirectly supervised	Level 4 Independent	
Recognise normal endometrium					
Recognise changes of endometrium with menstrual cycle					
Recognise atrophic endometrium					
Suspect malignant change in endometrium					
Recognise and categorise congenital uterine anomalies					
Recognise and categorise uterine fibroids					
Perform hysteroscopy post-endometrial resection/ablation					
Appropriate use of local anaesthetic for hysteroscopy					
Perform global and directed endometrial biopsy					
Recognise and treat endocervical lesions					
Locate and remove 'lost' intra-uterine contraceptive device					

Treatment modules

Within the above training framework, additional modules have been developed to allow hysteroscopists to plan treatment as well as diagnosis. The main entry criterion for these modules is that the individual should have successfully completed the diagnostic hysteroscopy module. The treatment modules cover subjects such as levonorgestrel intra-uterine system, using bipolar electrosurgery, and endometrial ablation.

For each module, the theoretical component may be taught over one day and it should include training on models and some live operating. The practical training should be undertaken in the trainees' base hospital under the direction of their trainers. The syllabus should include undertaking a set number of cases to

achieve competence at the 4 training levels outlined earlier. The trainee should produce some
case studies for assessment as well. The trainer
should be satisfied that the trainee is capable of
independent practice. Re-certification should
depend on case numbers, audit, and demonstra-
tion of continuous professional development.

A CURRICULUM FOR ADVANCED HYSTEROSCOPIC SURGERY TRAINING

The primary goal of this training is to produce
hysteroscopists who possess the knowledge,
technical skills, and attitudes required to
function as a qualified hysteroscopic surgeon
providing specialised ambulatory healthcare to
women with abnormal uterine bleeding *etc*.

Below, we describe a special skills training
module in advanced hysteroscopic surgery from
the UK. It can be adapted and modified to suite
the specification of training in a different country. The special skills are defined as specific
skills (clinical, teaching and managerial) that are
beyond those required for the acquisition of a
Certificate of Completion of General Gynaecology Training. In the UK, modules have been
developed, in conjunction with various specialist

Table 11.6 Syllabus of the special skill module in advanced hysteroscopy

- Generic clinical skills
- Diagnostic hysteroscopy
- Intra-uterine polyps
- Fibroids
- Endometrial resection/ablation
- Hysteroscopic complications
- Clinical audit

societies. The Royal College of Obstetrics and
Gynaecologists has developed a module in
advanced hysteroscopic surgery in collaboration with the British Society for Gynaecologic
Endoscopy. Trainees undertaking this module
are in an advanced stage of their general obstetrics and gynaecology training having completed
their core training. At this advanced stage,
trainees should have at least one, and preferably
two, clinical sessions a week dedicated to this
specialised hysteroscopic training. For the
majority of trainees, the modules outlined in
Table 11.6 should be completed within one year.

Table 11.7 Hysteroscopic special skills training programme requirements

1. Provide a service for the referral and transfer of patients who would benefit from the ambulatory specialised hysteroscopic facilities, expertise and experience

2. Have an adequate hysteroscopic workload providing a full range of experience in this field

3. Have established close collaboration with other gynaecologists within and outwith the centre, including major regional roles in continuing postgraduate education and training, audit, research, advice and co-ordination

4. Have a programme director who can co-ordinate the training programme and accept the responsibility for supervision of trainees

5. Have adequate library, laboratory and other resources to support learning, training and research needs, and to provide the resources for a research programme related to hysteroscopic training.

Table 11.8 Contents of theoretical advanced hysteroscopy course

Instrumentation and safety

Documentation

Analgesia

Electrosurgery

Distension media

Fluid management

Diagnosis and management of congenital uterine abnormalities

Diagnosis and management of Asherman syndrome

Transcervical resection of the endometrium following previous endometrial resection/ablation

Prevention and management of complications

Cervical trauma

Haemorrhage: primary and secondary

Fluid overload

Infection

Electrosurgical injury

New developments

Preceptors

The special skills training should be undertaken under the supervision of a preceptor. Preceptors must be actively involved in hysteroscopic surgery and be a member of the relevant Society for Gynaecological Endoscopy. As a general guideline, the person running the hysteroscopy service in the unit would be a suitable preceptor. Table 11.7 shows the requirements to be fulfilled by a special skills training programme. Preceptors will find this text helpful in planning their teaching programme. They should undertake direct supervision of the trainee for the bulk of the module. The preceptor should ensure the availability other professionals to cover their absence. It is the preceptor's duty to ensure that the professional to whom the duty of training is delegated is sufficiently competent, willing and able to teach the trainee. Dual preceptorship may be of some benefit to trainees. Preceptors should

sign off individual's skills competences, once they have been learnt by the trainee and demonstrated to the preceptor's satisfaction. A formal and regular trainee appraisal should be carried out.

Theoretical training

The knowledge component of training should be obtained by private study, under guidance of the preceptor using this book. In addition, the knowledge component will also be supplemented by the trainee's attendance at a theoretical course (Table 11.8) which should provide the essential knowledge component of training for this module. The importance of the Internet in education is well-recognised. Modern, Web-based learning provides the means for changing fundamentally the way in which instruction is delivered. A wealth of resources and techniques now exist which serve the purpose of teaching. This comes as a

Table 11.9 Generic skills of advanced hysteroscopic surgery

SKILL	Competence levels				Preceptor to sign and date when competence achieved
	Level 1 Observed	Level 2 Directly supervised	Level 3 Indirectly supervised	Level 4 Independent	
Counselling for procedure					
Assembling equipment					
Selection of appropriate equipment					
Patient positioning					
Orientation					
Safe dilatation of cervix					
Safe introduction of hysteroscope					
Safe use of energy sources					
Use of appropriate distension media					
Use of fluid management devices					
Management of vaso-vagal syndrome					
Excision of polyps using mechanical devices or bipolar electrodes					
Perform transcervical resection of polyps					
Appropriate use of priming agents, e.g. GnRH agonists					
Resect/ablate type 0 fibroid					
Resect/ablate type I fibroid					
Resect /ablate type II fibroid including two-stage procedures					
Treatment of small fibroids in the ambulatory care setting					

secondary pathway after successful completion of the practical training. Multimedia learning resources combined with CD-ROMs and workbooks attempt to explore the essential concepts of training by using the full power of multimedia which contains a plethora of hysteroscopy study material such as free downloads, hysteroscopic videos, animation, pictures, articles, updates and frequently asked questions with the help of leading hysteroscopists and interactive quizzes or even conduct advanced online surgical training through the Internet. These resources provide students with 'self-help' learning to complement a textbook such as this one.

Practical training

Every trainee should have the opportunity for an individual development and learning plan. There should be a named preceptor and a mentor who facilitates and helps provide a secure, confidential and supportive atmosphere to the trainee. This learning environment promotes the concentration of very specialised expertise. Hence, the trainees will learn the full range of outpatient hysteroscopic procedures under direct supervision including: flexible/rigid hysteroscopy and diagnostic/operative hysteroscopy. The practical component will involve attendance at ambulatory hysteroscopy clinics as well as theatre sessions where hysteroscopic procedures are undertaken. The trainee has to attend at least 30 such sessions and attendance must be documented. Trainees should attend 10 clinics where the counselling of women about hysteroscopic surgery, as well as alternatives, is undertaken. Trainees should complete a clinical audit on a subject related to the use of hysteroscopic surgery in the management of gynaecological conditions.

Completion of a logbook will allow the preceptor and trainee to monitor progress and identify deficiencies over the course of training. It is important to note that the logbook is a record of competence rather than experience. The preceptor and trainee should review the progress of training on a regular basis using four levels of competence outlined earlier. The trainee and preceptor should regularly discuss the management of cases. It is imperative that the trainee's progress meets standards that satisfy the preceptor and that the trainee can perform each exercise independently (Table 11.9).

Training is complete once all the competencies have been achieved, the audit has been assessed as being satisfactory by the preceptor, and a theoretical course has been attended. At this stage, the preceptor should sign the completion of training form. A certificate of completion of special skills training will then be issued. In the UK the certificate is issued jointly by The Royal College of Obstetrics and Gynaecology and the British Society for Gynaecological Endoscopy.

FUTURE DEVELOPMENT OF SUBSPECIALISATION

It has been suggested that the way forward is to develop advanced hysteroscopic surgery as a recognised subspecialisation. So far, there is no official accreditation of such a subspecialisation in hysteroscopy, but many individual clinicians have achieved the levels of excellence outlined in Table 11.10 through personal interest and training.

Table 11.10 The aim of a subspecialisation

1.	To improve knowledge, practice, teaching and research in the subspecialty
2.	To promote the concentration of very specialised expertise, special facilities and clinical material that will be of considerable benefit to some patients
3.	To establish a close understanding and working relationship with other disciplines involved in each of the subspecialty fields
4.	To encourage co-ordinated management of relevant clinical services throughout a region
5.	To accept a major regional responsibility for higher training, research and audit in the subspecialty fields
6.	To improve the recruitment of highly talented trainees into the recognised subspecialty

Key points

➢ Diagnostic hysteroscopy training should focus mainly on hysteroscopy as a diagnostic procedure. It can be undertaken by any interested professional – a nurse, a general practitioner or a gynaecologist.

➢ Advanced hysteroscopic surgery training should be particularly directed to gynaecologists either in training or qualified specialists. It should be delivered under the supervision of a preceptor to inculcate operative skills in an ambulatory setting.

➢ The knowledge component of training may be obtained by private study. In addition, the knowledge component may be supplemented by the attendance at a theoretical course.

➢ The practical training must involve attendance at ambulatory hysteroscopy clinics where competence in hysteroscopic procedures is gained through supervised training.

➢ Assessment of training should be competence-based. A trainee should be able to obtain an informal consent; recognise normal and abnormal findings; correlate the findings with the presenting symptoms, endocrine status or pathology; be competent in ambulatory hysteroscopic techniques; establish a diagnosis of hysteroscopic complications; formulate a plan of management; effectively communicate information to patients including discussion on alternatives; and be able to perform an audit of practice.

12 Answers to questions

OBJECTIVE: To provide correct answers to questions and an explanation for these answers.

CHAPTER 3

1. The flexible hysteroscope

Helps to overcome difficulties in viewing the cornual areas	True
Helps in entering acutely anteverted and retroverted uterus	True
Cannot be used in ambulatory setting	False
When compared with rigid hysteroscopy, it is believed to be associated with more pain	False

The flexible hysteroscope was developed to overcome difficulties in viewing the cornual areas and in entering acutely anteverted and retroverted uterus. It is a safe, successful, and reliable method of investigating abnormal uterine bleeding in ambulatory setting.

When compared with rigid hysteroscopy, flexible hysteroscopy is believed to be associated with less pain both at introduction of the hysteroscope and during the procedure itself especially when using the smaller diameter scope. However, flexible systems have not become wide-spread because of their high cost, fragility and difficulty in sterilisation.

2. Rigid hysteroscopes

Are available in different angles of vision ranging from 0° to 30°	True
Their external diameters vary from 5 mm to 7 mm	False
Magnification is inversely proportional to the distance of the object from the lens	True
Continuous liquid flow is indicated in patients with bleeding	True

Technical improvements aim at maintaining high resolution at various distances and with various magnifications. Rigid telescopes are available in different angles of vision ranging from 0° (180°) to 30° (150°, forward-oblique), the former being the most popular for ambulatory hysteroscopy. Their external diameters vary from 1.2 mm to 4 mm. Telescopes are focused at infinity; therefore, magnification is inversely proportional to the distance of the object from the lens. Double (continuous) flow system is indicated in patients with bleeding because it can maintain a clear vision.

3. Distension media

Carbon dioxide is a gas that is rapidly absorbed and cleared easily from the body by respiration	True
CO_2 can be used only in the inpatient setting	False
Shoulder tip pain is one of the disadvantages postoperatively	True
Air bubbles could obscure the view	True

Carbon dioxide is a colourless gas that is rapidly absorbed and cleared easily from the body by respiration. It can be used safely for outpatient hysteroscopic purposes. A steady flow of CO_2 allows even uterine cavity distension. In order to keep a safe and constant flow of CO_2, a pre-set hysteroflator, which automatically maintain pressure at between 100–120 mmHg, with a flow of 30–60 ml/min, should be used. The controlled flow of this gas keeps the intra-uterine pressure between 40–80 mmHg. With large quantities or uncontrolled delivery of CO_2, gas embolism can result in serious complications. The levels of CO_2 used during an entire hysteroscopic examination are far less than those that produce significant toxicity. Disadvantages include creation of air bubbles, which could obscure the view especially if there is bleeding, shoulder tip pain in some women due to gaseous irritation of the diaphragm and that it is not able to clear the uterine cavity of debris in comparison with fluid media.

4. Low viscosity distension media

Dextrose (5–10%), dextran (4–6%) and saline solutions all are low-viscosity distension media	True
They are considered suitable for the use of monopolar electric current	False
Normal saline is commonly used in office hysteroscopy	True
Comparing CO_2 and saline, both media are comparable in terms of overall patient discomfort, satisfaction and clarity of view	False

Low viscosity fluids such as dextrose (5–10%), dextran (4–6%) and saline solutions can be used to produce uterine distension for diagnostic purposes. However, as these solutions are electrolyte based, they are considered unsuitable for procedures that require the use of monopolar electric current. Normal saline is commonly used for uterine distension in office hysteroscopy. It is easily available at low cost. A randomised study comparing CO_2 with saline, as distension media for outpatient hysteroscopy, concluded that both media are comparable in terms of overall patient discomfort and satisfaction but saline provides superior views.

5. The Versascope

Is a small diameter hysteroscope (1.8 mm) in a disposable outer sheath of 3.5 mm	True
Contains a working channel for instruments up to 2 mm in diameter	True

Uses a monopolar electrode	False
Is very useful in ambulatory and office operative hysteroscopy	True

The Versacope is a semirigid hysteroscope for use in outpatient settings. A small diameter hysteroscope (1.8 mm), with a working length of 28 cm and a 0° lens, allows a field of view of 75°. A disposable outer sheath (continuous flow system) of 3.5 mm contains an expandable working channel for instruments up to 2 mm diameter (a disposable bipolar electrode). Energy is delivered from the generator to the tissue through the active electrode. This causes immediate cellular rupture and vaporisation. The energy then passes through the saline to the return electrode and back to the generator. It can cut, coagulate, vaporise and desiccate small intra-uterine lesions such as polyps, focal adhesions, small pedunculated submucous myoma, and small uterine septa.

This innovation is very useful in ambulatory operative hysteroscopy because the electrodes fit easily into the 5-Fr (1.6 mm) operating channel available on most hysteroscopes used for outpatient hysteroscopy.

CHAPTER 4

1. **In postmenopausal bleeding, what is the most likely diagnosis?**

Atrophic vaginitis	True
Endometrial polyp	False
Endometrial hyperplasia and carcinoma	False
Cervical polyp and cancer	False

Postmenopausal bleeding (PMB): is bleeding from the reproductive system that occurs 12 months or more after cessation of menstrual periods due to menopause. In 90% of cases, examination and investigation will find either no obvious cause or an innocent one. The commonest innocent cause is atrophic vaginitis. Cervical and endometrial polyps are further common findings with a 10–15% likelihood of endometrial pathology, particularly cancer. Endometrial adenocarcinoma accounts for 1.5–13.5% of patients with PMB.

2. **In the initial investigation of women with postmenopausal bleeding:**

Transvaginal ultrasound scan has a high sensitivity	True
Outpatient hysteroscopy is the investigation of choice	False
Magnetic resonance imaging (MRI) should be used if available	False
Pelvic examination can be replaced by transvaginal ultrasound scan	False

In evaluating a woman with postmenopausal bleeding, the sensitivity of transvaginal ultrasound as a test for the detection of endometrial pathology is high (94–100%). The variation in the sensitivity depends on the cut-off point used for endometrial thickness (*i.e.* < 4 mm or < 5 mm). It has an virtually 100% negative predictive value; therefore, a normal value eliminates the need for further investigation. Only when the endometrial thickness is above the cut-off value is hysteroscopy or further assessment indicated. Magnetic resonance imaging (MRI) scans can be used for the staging of endometrial cancer; however, its role is still unclear. At the present time, MRI has no role in the investigation of postmenopausal bleeding. As an initial investigation of postmenopausal bleeding, outpatient hysteroscopy is considered to be too invasive. This is particularly the case when one considers the sensitivity and specificity of ultrasound (*see* Chapter 9). The ultrasound scan must be preceded by a vaginal examination to exclude cervical pathology.

3.   In postmenopausal bleeding:

Outpatient endometrial biopsy is often necessary	True
A pelvic ultrasound scan is performed for endometrial thickness measurement and adnexal masses	True
Outpatient hysteroscopy allows direct visualisation of the uterine cavity	True
Inpatient dilatation and curettage is required routinely	False

In postmenopausal bleeding, the aim of all investigations is to exclude gynaecological cancer. Therefore, outpatient endometrial biopsy is often necessary to obtain an endometrial sample for histological assessment. Current evidence suggests that an endometrial thickness of < 4 mm reduces the likelihood of endometrial cancer substantially. Ovarian tumours can present as postmenopausal bleeding, but rarely. Outpatient hysteroscopy allows direct visualisation of the uterine cavity, which is particularly useful for excluding endometrial polyps or fibroids. Inpatient hysteroscopy is required only if the outpatient assessment is either inadequate or impossible to perform.

4.   In obtaining consent for hysteroscopic procedure:

The consent should be obtained by any member of the team	False
Clinicians do not breach confidentiality when they disclose information with their patients' consent	True
Patients should give separate consent for information about them to be shared among healthcare professionals	False
The valid consent of a competent patient can only be given by the patient	True

The consent should be obtained by the clinician who will be performing the hysteroscopic procedure. A recent study of informed consent suggests that patients may be asked for their consent from a doctor who has little knowledge or experience of the procedure in question. In this study many doctors said that their major problem in gaining informed consent from patients for procedures was their own lack of knowledge and experience of specific procedures and the risks involved. In addition, they often obtained consented for procedures they will not carry out themselves. The results of the study show that many doctors were uncertain of the elements that are required if consent is to be both informed and legally valid. Hence, the consent should be obtained by the clinician who will perform the procedure. Clinicians must convey to patients the reality and necessity of information sharing within health teams without obtaining consent *per se*. The last statement is self-explanatory.

5. **When making video recordings of hysteroscopy:**

Clinicians do not need to take consent for it   False

Withholding permission will not affect the quality of care patients receive   True

Using recordings for purposes outside the scope of the original consent needs
further consent   True

Patients should understand that recordings are given the same level of protection as
medical records against improper disclosure   True

When making recordings, clinicians must seek permission to make the recording and obtain consent to use the recording made for reasons other than the patient's treatment or assessment (recordings made for the training or assessment of doctors, audit, research or medicolegal reasons). Clinicians should also ensure that patients are under no pressure to give their permission for the recording to be made and that withholding permission will not affect the quality of care they receive. After the recording, patients should understand that recordings are given the same level of protection as medical records against improper disclosure.

CHAPTER 5

1. **Regarding the innervations of the uterine body and uterine cervix:**

The presacral space begins at the bifurcation of the aorta into the iliac arteries   True

Lying on the coccyx, with the middle sacral vessels, is the pelvic autonomic
nervous system   False

The inferior hypogastric nerve plexus is a collection of nerves lying just lateral to the
ovaries in the infundibulopelvic ligaments   False

This plexus contains sympathetic pelvic splanchnic nerves from the thoracolumbar
trunk and parasympathetics from the craniosacral trunk   True

The innervations of the uterine body and uterine cervix is best understood by reviewing the anatomical features of the neural network in the pelvis. The presacral space begins at the bifurcation of the aorta into the iliac arteries. Lying on the sacrum (not the coccyx), with the middle sacral vessels, is the pelvic autonomic nervous system, the presacral nerve plexus (or the superior hypogastric plexus). It divides into two nerves, the right and left hypogastric nerves that lead to the inferior hypogastric nerve plexus. This collection of nerves lies just lateral to the uterus and vagina in the uterosacral/cardinal ligament complex. This plexus contains sympathetic pelvic splanchnic nerves from the thoracolumbar trunk and para-sympathetics from the craniosacral trunk. It has three portions: (i) the vesical anterior plexus; (ii) the uterovaginal plexus (also known as Frankenhauser's or Lee-Frankenhauser's plexus); and (iii) the middle rectal plexus.

2. **Regarding Frankenhauser's plexus:**

It innervates the lower part of the uterine body, the cervix, and the upper vagina   True

It lies on the dorso-medial surface of the uterine vessels, just lateral to the uterosacral/cardinal ligament complex	True
The uterine vessels, within the cardinal ligaments, enter the cervix at the 3- and 9-o'clock positions	True
All of the innervation of the uterine body is truly from Frankenhauser's plexus	False

It is Frankenhauser's plexus that appears to innervate lower part of the uterine body, the cervix, and the upper vagina. It lies on the dorso-medial surface of the uterine vessels, just lateral to the uterosacral/cardinal ligament complex. The uterine vessels, within the cardinal ligaments, enter the cervix at the 3- and 9-o'clock positions. An additional set of nerves may also be contained within the uterosacral complex that insert at 4- and 8-o'clock position on the posterior aspect of the uterus. It has been debated whether all of the innervation of the uterine body is truly from Frankenhauser's plexus. Other possibilities include collateral neural connections from of the infundibulo-pelvic ligament, which contains the ovarian neurovascular bundle. This may be particularly true as it relates to the uterine body.

3. **Regarding pain and discomfort during hysteroscopy:**

Distension of the uterine cavity causes discomfort and pain	True
The higher the distension pressure in the uterus the more the discomfort	True
A minimum of 60 mmHg is needed to separate the uterine walls	False
The size of hysteroscope and sheath has no impact on pain and success rates	False

Distension of the uterine cavity causes discomfort and pain. The lower the distension pressure in the uterus the less the discomfort: a minimum of 30 mmHg is needed to separate the uterine walls. In the outpatient setting, the pressure should be kept to this minimum and increased only if the view is poor. The size of hysteroscope and sheath has an impact on pain and success rates. Diameters of less than 3.5 mm are well tolerated in the outpatient setting. Addition of endometrial biopsy to hysteroscopy increases pain.

4. **Additional contributing factors to the pain:**

Addition of endometrial biopsy to hysteroscopy increases pain	True
Menopause has an impact on the procedure being painful	False
Talking to the patient is a recognised factor in distracting women's attention during the procedure	True
Irrespective of the distension medium used, pelvic discomfort is worse in nulliparous women than in multiparous women	True

The International Association for the Study of Pain gives this definition: 'pain is an unpleasant sensory and emotional experience associated with actual or potential tissue damage'. Irrespective of the distension medium used, pelvic discomfort is worse in nulliparous women than in multiparous women. The size of hysteroscope and sheath has an impact on pain and success rates. Diameters of less than 3.5 mm are well tolerated in the outpatient setting. Addition of endometrial biopsy to hysteroscopy increases pain. Menopause has no effect on the procedure being painful. Talking to the patient during the procedure distracts them and allows them to focus on other subjects, hence the role of a well trained nurse (an auxiliary healthcare assistant).

5. Regarding pain control in outpatient hysteroscopy:

The application of topical anaesthetic agents has a significant benefit	False
The deep paracervical block is of unproven efficacy	False
Analgesia, in the form of paracetamol and/or NSAIDs, may effectively be used for ambulatory hysteroscopic procedures	True
Vaginoscopy means passing the hysteroscope through the internal cervical os without speculum or volsellum	True

Because the neurophysiology of the uterus is complex and not entirely understood, the ability to find new and effective means to provide anaesthesia to the uterus has been challenging. The majority of outpatient diagnostic hysteroscopy cases do not need anaesthesia if small diameter instruments are used. Usually, anaesthesia/analgesia is only necessary during outpatient operative hysteroscopy if needing to dilate the cervix. The application of topical anaesthetic agents appears to have little or no added benefit for endometrial procedures, but can make the application of the tenaculum more comfortable for the patient. The deep injection technique for paracervical block provides most consistent pain relief. Analgesia, in the form of paracetamol and/or diclofenac may effectively be used for ambulatory hysteroscopic procedures. Vaginoscopy is an approach that may eliminate patient discomfort related to the traditional approach. One of its key steps is to pass the hysteroscope through the internal cervical os without speculum or volsellum.

6. Ambulatory hysteroscopy

Is associated with severe pain in less than 10% of women	True
Has a failure rate of 8% of all attempted procedures	False
Anaesthesia is only required if there is a need to dilate the cervix	True
When using bipolar energy to remove polyps or treat fibroids, anaesthesia is essential	False

Outpatient hysteroscopy stimulates visceral pain; however, with proper pre-operative patient counselling and good technique, most women find the procedure acceptable. Some 3–10% of women undergoing the procedure experience severe pain. The failure rate of ambulatory hysteroscopy is about 4% and is most commonly due to anatomical factors such as cervical stenosis. It is important to remember that the majority of outpatient diagnostic hysteroscopy cases do not need any anaesthesia or analgesia. It is only required if there is a need to overcome cervical stenosis, *i.e.* to dilate the cervix or during outpatient operative hysteroscopy. One can remove polyps, or treat fibroids with minimal pain when using bipolar energy, snares or mechanical instruments.

CHAPTER 6

1. **Indications for outpatient hysteroscopy include:**

Resection of type II submucous fibroids	False
Diagnosis of uterine synechiae	True
Location and retrieval of lost or misplaced intrauterine contraceptive device	True
Transcervical resection of the endometrium for menorrhagia	False

Submucous fibroids, types 0 and type I, distorting the uterine cavity are well placed for hysteroscopic diagnosis and removal. Most authors recommend removal of fibroids no more than 2 cm in diameter in the outpatient setting. Outpatient hysteroscopy is ideal for the detection of intra-uterine adhesions. Treatment can be offered using mechanical instruments or a bipolar twizzle electrode in the outpatient setting.

2. **Abnormal uterine bleeding:**

Is the commonest reason for hysteroscopic examination	True
Abnormal uterine bleeding accounts for more than 50% of referrals to the gynaecologist	False
Structural lesions responsible for abnormal uterine bleeding are often at their peak during the postmenopausal period	False
Between 5–10% of all women with postmenopausal bleeding will have endometrial cancer	True

Abnormal uterine bleeding is the commonest reason for hysteroscopic examination. It accounts for more than 20% of referrals to the gynaecologist and for 25% of gynaecological procedures in premenstrual women. Structural lesions responsible for abnormal uterine bleeding are often at their peak during the perimenopausal period. Between 5–10% of all women with postmenopausal bleeding will have endometrial cancer.

3. **In the investigation of infertility:**

Outpatient hysteroscopy is used routinely	False
Hysteroscopy has a high false-positive rate due to distortion of the uterine cavity from mucus, debris, and blood	False
Outpatient hysteroscopy is the diagnostic procedure of choice in diagnosing intra-uterine anomalies in infertile patients	True
Outpatient hysteroscopy has a sensitivity of 85% in detecting tubal pathology	False

Hysteroscopy is not used routinely in the investigation of infertility. It is more common to use hysterosalpingography. Hysterosalpingography (not hysteroscopy) has a high false positive rate due to transient distortion of the uterine cavity from mucus, debris, bubbles and blood. Hysterosalpingography (not hysteroscopy) has 85–100% sensitivity in detecting tubal pathology in infertile patients but only 44% sensitivity in documented intra-uterine malformations and 75% in intra-uterine adhesions (synechiae). Outpatient hysteroscopy is the diagnostic procedure of choice in confirming and planning treatment for intra-uterine anomalies in infertile patients. It also permits the inspection of the cervical canal and the tubal ostia. Lesions detected by outpatient hysteroscopy in infertility investigations include endometrial polyps, submucous fibroids, intra-uterine adhesions (synechiae), and uterine septa.

4. **In infertility:**

Of women presenting with infertility, 20% have endometrial polyps	False
There is good evidence that women with polyps have a higher rate of spontaneous miscarriage	False
The value of routine hysteroscopic removal of these polyps before fertility treatment is unknown	True
There is evidence to show that fibroids directly affect fertility	False

Of women presenting with infertility, 10% have endometrial polyps. There has been some suggestion that women with polyps have a higher rate of spontaneous miscarriage but there is no evidence of lower pregnancy rates in this group. Outpatient hysteroscopy easily identifies women with sub-fertility and endometrial polyps but the value of routine hysteroscopic removal of these polyps before fertility treatment is unknown. Fibroids have rarely been shown to be a direct cause of infertility. There is evidence to show that fibroids indirectly affect fertility because they alter the contractility of the uterus and may disrupt normal sperm migration. Fibroids may also affect the vascular and molecular profiles of sites of implantation and, in some cases, cause partial obstruction of the tubal ostia.

5. **Absolute contra-indications to outpatient hysteroscopy include:**

Recent uterine perforation	False
Pregnancy	False
Cervical cancer	True
Heavy uterine bleeding	True

Only cervical cancer and heavy uterine bleeding are absolute contra-indications to outpatient hysteroscopy.

CHAPTER 7

1. **Indications for ambulatory operative hysteroscopy**

Targeted biopsy under direct vision	True
Most experts would recommend that polyps of up to 5 cm in diameter can be removed	False

Most experts would recommend that type 0, type I and type II submucous fibroids can all be treated in the outpatient setting	False
In the majority of cases of lost IUDs, the device is still present in the uterine cavity	True

Focal lesions in the endometrium, which are suspicious or look abnormal, are best biopsied using a targeted approach. Providing the hysteroscope has an operative channel then the surgeon can, under direct vision, take tissue samples from the area. Most experts would recommend that polyps of < 3 cm in diameter can be removed this way. Larger polyps take longer and are best managed by resection under general or regional anaesthesia. Submucous fibroids can be classified as:

Type 0 – 100% of the fibroid is within the endometrial cavity

Type I – > 50% is within the uterine cavity

Type II – < 50% is within the uterine cavity

Most experts would recommend that only type 0 and type I submucous fibroids of < 2 cm in diameter should be treated in the outpatient setting. In the majority of cases of lost IUDs, the device is still present in the uterine cavity with its thread curled up into the uterine cavity out of view on speculum examination.

2. Intra-uterine adhesions

Result from trauma in the postpartum or post-abortal period	True
Generally lead to menorrhagia	False
Moderate adhesions are fibromuscular, thick and avascular	False
Severe adhesions are likely to bleed on division	False

Intra-uterine adhesions result from trauma in the postpartum or postabortal period. It generally leads to hypomenorrhoea or amenorrhoea. Hysteroscopy is effective in evaluating the uterine cavity and outlining the precise distortion that exists from the adhesions and also permitting direct treatment. The extent of the adhesions varies from focal to multiple areas. The extent also determines the prognosis. Adhesions are classified as mild, moderate or severe. When mild, they are filmy, thin and usually only of recent occurrence, and are easily amenable to outpatient hysteroscopic division either by mechanical instruments or by electrosurgical methods. They have a better prognosis than the moderate or severe varieties. Moderate adhesions are fibromuscular, thick and covered by endometrium and may bleed on division. Severe adhesions are usually composed of connective tissue only, without endometrial covering and are unlikely to bleed on division as they are more fibrotic.

3. Division of uterine septa

25% of women with a septate uterus have recurrent pregnancy loss	True
The septa are poorly vascularised making them ideal for hysteroscopic division	True

| Hysteroscopic division yields low success rates | False |
| Caesarean section is mandatory should pregnancy be carried to term | False |

Of women with a septate uterus, 25% have recurrent pregnancy loss. The septa are poorly vascularised making them ideal for hysteroscopic division. Every effort should be made to ensure a thick covering of myometrium at the uterine fundus (transvaginal scan). If this is not certain then the division is best carried out under laparoscopic control to maintain uniform transillumination of the fundal portion of the uterus while the septum is divided. Hysteroscopic division offers high success rates and avoids the increased morbidity from abdominal operation and is more cost effective and avoids the risk of postoperative intra-abdominal adhesions. Following hysteroscopic division, successful pregnancy rates of 85–90% have been quoted in some series. Generally, patients are advised to delay pregnancy for at least 4–6 weeks. Caesarean section is not mandatory should pregnancy be carried to term.

4. **Outpatient endometrial ablation**

The approved devices have patient satisfaction rates of more than 80%	True
With microwave endometrial ablation (MEA) failure is more likely to occur when the uterine cavity is greater than 12 cm	True
MEA can be used when intra-uterine fibroids exist	True
Endometrial priming is an absolute requirement	False

The ablative devices more suited for the outpatient setting are the second generation, so-called, global endometrial ablation devices. There have been many innovative devices proposed for achieving rapid, simple global endometrial ablation. The overall success rate of all these various devices is more than 80%. Of these, the microwave endometrial ablation was the only device initially licensed for use in patients with submucous fibroids up to 3 cm diameter or uterine cavity depth of up to 14 cm. Hydro ThermAblator™ (HTA) can also be used. Cavities of > 11 cm have a higher chance of treatment failure. Women who have had lower segment caesarean section can be treated providing the scar thickness measured by ultrasound scan is > 8 mm. Endometrial priming is not absolutely mandatory.

5. **Essure™**

Essure hysteroscopic sterilisation is 99.8% effective in preventing pregnancy after 3 years' follow-up	True
It takes up to 45 minutes to perform	False
Has a high patient satisfaction rating	True
An alternative method of contraception must be used for 3 months after the procedure	True

Essure™ developed by Conceptus Inc. is a new system that tries to achieve permanent contraception via outpatient hysteroscopic sterilisation. In the early studies, bilateral tubal occlusion was demonstrated in 96% of cases and 6 months follow-up confirmed bilateral occlusion in all patients. Essure is 99.80% effective in preventing pregnancy after 3 years of follow-up. It can be performed in 15–35 minutes and has a high patient satisfaction rating. An alternative method of contraception must be used for 3 months.

CHAPTER 8

1. **Ambulatory hysteroscopy:**

Is generally a safe procedure	True
In diagnostic procedures, most complications are rare and seldom life-threatening	True
Complications of ambulatory operative procedures are mainly due to fluid intravasation	False
The operator's experience is irrelevant to complications	False

Ambulatory hysteroscopy is a safe procedure by any standard. Complications can occur when inappropriate instruments or techniques are used. Most complications of hysteroscopy are rare; if they do occur, they are seldom life-threatening particularly in diagnostic procedures. Ambulatory operative procedures tend to be short in duration and, as the patient is awake and responsive to painful stimuli, the chances are that fluid intravasation problems are unlikely and difficult procedure will be abandoned soon due to patient intolerability minimising risk of complications. Some of the complications are entry-related, so avoid dilating the cervix unnecessarily and always introduce the hysteroscope under direct vision. Other complications are related to surgeons' experience and type of procedure.

2. **Complications of operative hysteroscopy:**

Are related to the type of procedure	True
False passage is the most common complication	True
Hysteroscopic polypectomy and resection of fibroids are associated with high rates of complications	False
Resection of uterine septa has significantly higher complication rates than polypectomy	True

Operative hysteroscopic procedures are more risky, with uterine perforation being the most common complication. Uterine perforation is a rare event. A recent Royal College of Obstetricians and Gynaecologists' guideline of taking consent for diagnostic hysteroscopy under general anaesthetic quoted a figure as low as 8/1000 for uterine perforation. For ambulatory procedures, the figure is much lower. In a large systematic review of studies of over 25,000 women only 4 cases (1/6000) of uterine perforations occurred. Hysteroscopic polypectomy is associated with lower rates of complications (12 times lower than synechiolysis). Among other hysteroscopic procedures, resection of fibroids and uterine septa have significantly higher rates of complications (4–7 times higher operative complications than polypectomy) mainly due to fluid intravasation.

3. **Complications of excessive absorption of distension media:**

With hysteroscopic procedures, occur equally in ambulatory and inpatient settings	False
Should be extremely rare if the correct insufflator (hysteroflator) is used	True
Cardiac arrhythmias do not occur with diagnostic hysteroscopy using CO_2	False
Gas embolism during hysteroscopy is rare but fatal	True

Complications produced by the distension media are specific to hysteroscopic surgery though it also occurs in endoscopic prostatic procedures. The problems are less likely in ambulatory procedures. It is essential that all operating room staff are familiar with the side effects of the absorption of distension media and that responsibility for fluid balance is taken by a designated member of staff. Cardiac arrhythmia can occur even with diagnostic hysteroscopy using CO_2. The complication should be extremely rare if the correct insufflator is used. The hysteroflator delivers CO_2 at a rate of not more than 100 ml/min whereas the laparoflator can deliver 1–6 litres in the same time. A laparoflator should never be used for hysteroscopy. It is rare for CO_2 to produce any side effects if gas embolism of less than 400 ml occurs. Gas embolism during hysteroscopy is rare but can sometimes be rapidly fatal. Symptomatic gas embolism can occur when undissolved gas (air, CO_2) accumulates in the heart and/or pulmonary arteries compromising circulation and causing serious shock or death. Air embolism can occur when using bipolar diathermy in ambulatory operative hysteroscopy. Suspicion should arise when the patient suddenly gasps for air, with impalpable pulse, tonic convulsions, consciousness loss and cardiac arrest. Heart sounds suggesting intracardiac gas may be heard (Mill wheel murmur). The importance of monitoring for a rapid diagnosis and treatment remarkably improves the outcome. Immediate cardiopulmonary resuscitation is required until the crash team arrives and the patient is admitted to the intensive care unit. The diagnosis may be confirmed by aspiration of foamy blood from the central venous line, which is diagnostic and therapeutic at the same time.

4. **Fluids as distension media:**

Electrolytic solutions (normal saline or lactated Ringer's) can be used in conjunction with monopolar electrosurgical devices	False
Electrolytic solutions (normal saline or lactated Ringer's) can be used in conjunction with laser or bipolar energy	True
Glycine is used in conjunction with monopolar electrosurgical energy	True
Complications of dextran include coagulation disorders	True

Electrolytic solutions are capable of conducting electricity; therefore, they cannot be used in conjunction with monopolar electrosurgical devices. Recommended by the American Association of Gynecologic Laparoscopists (AAGL) for use in diagnostic cases and in operative cases in which mechanical instruments, laser or bipolar energy is used. Non-electrolytic solutions (glycine 1.5%, mannitol 5%) eliminate problems with electrical conductivity, and can be used in conjunction with monopolar energy but can increase the risk to patients of hyponatraemia and other complications. Complications of dextran include coagulation disorders, allergic reactions and adult respiratory distress syndrome.

5. **Prevention of fluid extravasation can be accomplished by:**

Using appropriate distension media and delivery systems	True
Keeping operating times to a minimum	True
Keeping fluid pressures as low as possible	True
Meticulous fluid balance. The procedure must be abandoned if the deficit rises to 2000 ml	False

Prevention can be accomplished by using appropriate distension media and delivery systems, keeping operating times to a minimum, keeping fluid pressures as low as possible because of fluid absorption if it exceeds venous pressure and by meticulous fluid balance. The procedure must be abandoned if the deficit rises to 750–1000 ml.

6. **Uterine perforation:**

In the British Mistletoe study, perforation occurred in 6/100 cases	False
Uterine perforation in ambulatory hysteroscopy is a rare event	True
Should be avoided by always introducing the telescope under direct vision	True
Laparoscopy should always be performed to exclude bleeding	False

Uterine perforation is a rare event. A recent Royal College of Obstetricians and Gynaecologists' guideline of taking consent for diagnostic hysteroscopy under general anaesthetic quoted a figure as low as 8/1000 for uterine perforation. For ambulatory procedures the figure is much lower. In a large systematic review of studies of over 25,000 women only 4 cases (1/6000) of uterine perforations occurred. Even for inpatient operative procedures, the incidence is low. In the British Mistletoe study, perforation occurred in 6/1000 and 6/1000 of cases, respectively, with roller ball and laser but in 13/1000 and 25/1000 of cases when roller ball and loop or loop alone were used. The uterus may be perforated by a dilator, the hysteroscope or an energy source. The management will depend on the size, site of the perforation, and whether there is risk of injury to another organ. Perforation occurs more frequently at the level of the fundus without significant bleeding and should be suspected if the dilator passes to a depth greater than the length of the uterine cavity. Perforation with the hysteroscope should be avoided by always introducing the telescope under direct vision. Simple perforation rarely causes any further damage and may be treated conservatively by admission, observation and appropriate broad-spectrum antibiotics. Laparoscopy may be considered to exclude bleeding. Complex perforation may be made with mechanical or electrical instruments and, therefore, may be associated with thermal injury to adjacent structures including bowel or large vessels. However, energy sources used in outpatient setting are usually bipolar energy (Versapoint), or heat (Thermachoice) that offer reduction of energy spread through the tissue during the procedure. If perforation is suspected, the energy source should be switched off and the hysteroscope left *in situ* while preparing for laparoscopy. Laparoscopic examination to exclude bowel injury may be all that is necessary. However, in the majority of cases of electrical injury and in all cases where laser has been used, laparotomy and detailed examination of the bowel, pelvic blood vessels and aorta is mandatory.

7. **Delayed complications of ambulatory hysteroscopy:**

Infection, vaginal discharge, adhesion formation and haemorrhage are all delayed complications of ambulatory hysteroscopy	False
Acute pelvic inflammatory disease is rare following hysteroscopic surgery	True
Vaginal discharge is common after any ablative procedure	True
Vaginal discharge can sometimes be prolonged (2–3 months)	False

An incidence of 2/1000 of infection has been reported in over 4000 diagnostic hysteroscopies. Acute pelvic inflammatory disease is rare following hysteroscopic surgery. The diagnosis is made by the presentation of the classic symptoms and signs and treatment should be by appropriate antibiotics following culture of vaginal swabs and blood (both aerobic and anaerobic). Vaginal discharge is common after any ablative procedure and can sometimes be prolonged (2–3 weeks); however, it is usually self-limiting. Patients should alert their healthcare provider if the vaginal discharges become offensive or if she develops pyrexia, heavy bleeding or severe lower abdominal pain.

CHAPTER 9

1. **You are asked to see a patient with 3 months' history of postmenopausal bleeding. Physical examination does not reveal any abnormality. The patient has heard that she may have polyps. Read the following abstract and answer the subsequent questions about this patient.**

ABSTRACT

Study objective: To assess the diagnostic potential of ultrasound in identifying polyps in postmenopausal bleeding.

Design: Prospective evaluation.

Setting: Outpatient ultrasound and hysteroscopy department of a university-affiliated hospital.

Patients: Two hundred women with an endometrial thickness assessment on ultrasound and in menopause for at least 1 year.

Interventions: Transvaginal ultrasound and office hysteroscopy, with eye-directed biopsy specimens obtained with a 5-mm, continuous-flow operative hysteroscope, and performed without anaesthesia. Hysteroscopy served as the 'gold' standard for diagnosis of polyps.

Measurements and main results: Endometrial polyps were seen on hysteroscopy in 35 women. Among 150 women, the endometrium was regular with thickness less than 4 mm. Of these, 15 had endometrial polyps. Among 50 women, the endometrium was irregular and/or thickness was 4 mm or more. Of these, 20 had endometrial polyps.

Conclusion: Hysteroscopy allows a proper diagnosis of endometrial polyps.

Now answer the following questions about this patient.

1 (i) Before performing any investigations, what is the probability that there is an endometrial polyp?
    This question is answered by finding out the proportion of women with polyps in the study sample.

    A.   about 1.75%

    B.   about 17.5%

    C.   about 20%

    D.   virtually 100%   **The correct answer is: B**

Endometrial polyps were seen on hysteroscopy in 35 out of the 200 women. This is equal to 17.5%.

1 (ii) An ultrasound examination has been carried out that shows endometrial thickness of more than 4 mm. What is the probability that there is an endometrial polyp?

    E.   virtually 100%

    F.   about 4%

    G.   about 20%

    H.   about 40%   **The correct answer is: H**

50 women had an endometrium that was irregular and/or thick > 4 mm or more. Of these, 20 had endometrial polyps. Giving a 40% probability of having endometrial polyps.

1 (iii) A student asks you to show how a 2 x 2 table (shown below) can be generated comparing ultrasound and hysteroscopic diagnosis.

	Hysteroscopy:polyp	Hysteroscopy:no polyp	
Ultrasound positive	True positive (TP)	False positive (FP)	TP+FP
Ultrasound negative	False negative (FN)	True negative (TN)	FN+TN
	TP+FN	FP+TN	Total

Which one of the following 4 tables fits the data presented in the paper?

Table A

	Hysteroscopy:polyp	Hysteroscopy:no polyp	
Ultrasound positive	20	30	50
Ultrasound negative	135	15	150
	155	45	200 patients

Table B

	Hysteroscopy:polyp	Hysteroscopy:no polyp	
Ultrasound positive	20	15	35
Ultrasound negative	30	135	160
	50	150	200 patients

Table C

	Hysteroscopy:polyp	Hysteroscopy:no polyp	
Ultrasound positive	20	30	50
Ultrasound negative	15	135	150
	35	165	200 patients

Table D

	Hysteroscopy:polyp	Hysteroscopy:no polyp	
Ultrasound positive	15	30	45
Ultrasound negative	20	135	155
	35	165	200 patients

The correct table is: C.

Endometrial polyps were seen on hysteroscopy in 35 women. Among 150 women, the endometrium was regular with thickness less than 4 mm (negative scan). Of these, 15 (false negative) had endometrial polyps. Among 50 women, the endometrium was irregular and/or thickness was 4 mm or more (positive scan). Of these, 20 had endometrial polyps (true positive).

1 (iv) You perform a hysteroscopy. Your view of the entire cavity is satisfactory. You see both tubal ostea clearly. You find normal-looking endometrium without any irregularities. You do not see any polyps. In the light of your findings:

A. You must arrange for the patient to have hysteroscopy and curettage under anaesthesia.

B. You can re-assure the patient that there are no polyps.

The correct answer is: B

As the hysteroscopy is the gold standard for endometrial polyp detection, with negative hysteroscopy you can re-assure the woman and discharge her.

2. **You are asked to see a 64-year-old patient with postmenopausal bleeding. Physical examination does not reveal any abnormality. Regarding endometrial cancer, read the following abstract and answer the following questions about this patient.**

ABSTRACT

Study objectives: The fundamental objective of this study was to determine the true value of hysteroscopy in the assessment of women with post-menopausal bleeding, namely in the diagnosis/exclusion of endometrial carcinoma.

Study methods: 158 women with post menopausal bleeding were studied with a rigid hysteroscope of 6 mm in external diameter for diagnostic purpose and for biopsy under direct vision. The uterine cavity was distended with CO_2 gas insufflations. Only a paracervical block with lidocaine was used. In all 158 cases, a biopsy was performed and the 'hysteroscopic diagnosis' was compared with the histological diagnosis. True and false positives as well as true and false negatives were calculated and, subsequently, the sensitivity, specificity, negative and positive predictive values, and overall efficiency were all evaluated. Prevalence is also indicated.

Results: The mean age of the women was 64.2 years, with a range of 40–83 years. We found 14 cases of endometrial carcinoma. The prevalence was 8.8%. 14 true positives, 17 false positives, 126 true negatives and 1 false negative were obtained. From the 17 false positives, 4 had a histological diagnosis of simple hyperplasia with cysts, 5 of glandular hyperplasia, and 8 had a normal histology. The false negative had a 'hysteroscopic diagnosis' of endometrial hyperplasia.

Conclusions: Our results show hysteroscopy to be a method with good sensitivity (93.3%), good overall efficiency (88.6%), and an excellent negative predictive value (99.2%). The specificity was 88.1%, and the positive predictive value was 45.1%. Because of the 'hysteroscopic diagnosis' of the false negative, we can conclude that the negative predictive value was virtually 100%.

Now answer the following questions about this patient.

2 (i)   Before performing hysteroscopy, what is the probability that there is endometrial cancer?

    A.   about 8.8%

    B.   about 88.6%

    C.   about 45.1%

    D.   virtually 100%   **The correct answer is: A**

This question is answered by finding out the prevalence of cancer in the study sample.

2 (ii) A student asks you to show how a 2 x 2 table (shown below) can be generated comparing hysteroscopy and histological diagnosis.

	Histology:cancer	Histology:not cancer	
Hysteroscopy positive	True positive (TP)	False positive (FP)	TP+FP
Hysteroscopy negative	False negative (FN)	True negative (TN)	FN+TN
	TP+FN	FP+TN	Total

Which one of the 4 tables fits the data presented in the paper?

Table A

	Histology:cancer	Histology:not cancer	
Hysteroscopy positive	126	17	143
Hysteroscopy negative	1	14	15
	127	143	158 patients

Table B

	Histology:cancer	Histology:not cancer	
Hysteroscopy positive	1	17	18
Hysteroscopy negative	14	126	140
	15	143	158 patients

Table C

	Histology:cancer	Histology:not cancer	
Hysteroscopy positive	14	17	31
Hysteroscopy negative	1	126	127
	15	143	158 patients

Table D

	Histology:cancer	Histology:not cancer	
Hysteroscopy positive	14	1	15
Hysteroscopy negative	17	126	143
	31	127	158 patients

    The correct table is: C.

The answer can be obtained from the Results section of the study sample.

2 (iii) You perform a hysteroscopy. Your findings reveal increased endometrial thickness, abnormal vascularisation, and irregularities. You are concerned that the patient might have cancer. In light of your findings, you arrange for the patient to have hysteroscopy and curettage under anaesthesia.

What is the probability that cancer will be present on histology?

A.   17/31

B.   126/127

C.   14/31

D.   1/127   **The correct answer is: C**

This question is answered by examining the number of women with positive hysteroscopy who had cancer.

2 (iv) If the hysteroscopy were negative, what would be the probability of missing a cancer?

A.   17/31

B.   126/127

C.   14/31

D.   1/127   **The correct answer is: D**

This question is answered by examining the number of women with negative hysteroscopy who had cancer.

3.   **You are asked to see a patient with postmenopausal bleeding for 3 months. Physical examination does not reveal any abnormality. The patient has heard that she may have cancer of the lining of the womb. Read the following abstracts, consider the information below, and answer the questions about this patient.**

ABSTRACT 1

Study of: Transvaginal sonography and progesterone challenge for identifying endometrial pathology in postmenopausal women.

Objective: To evaluate the usefulness of transvaginal sonographic (TVS) measurement of endometrial thickness for identifying endometrial pathology in postmenopausal women.

Methods: 284 postmenopausal women were examined by TVS: 130 asymptomatic women (group A) and 154 with uterine bleeding (group B). Endometrial thickness > 5 mm was considered pathological. All women with abnormal endometrium from group A and all women from group B underwent D&C.

Results: 107 patients from group B had abnormal sonographic and histological findings – benign (hyperplasia, polyp) or malignant (endometrial cancer). There was no cancer in cases with endometrial thickness <= 6 mm. The sensitivity and specificity of TVS for detecting endometrial pathology were 99% and 59%, respectively, if the cut-off limit of 5 mm was used.

Conclusion: TVS is a simple, well-tolerated, safe and reliable method for identifying endometrial pathology in postmenopausal women.

Consider the following information and definitions used in diagnostic studies:

2 x 2 table

	Hysteroscopy or ultrasound		
	Test result positive	Test result negative	
Histology cancer	True positive (TP)	False positive (FP)	TP+FP
Histology benign	False negative (FN)	True negative (TN)	FN+TN
	TP+FN	FP+TN	Total

Sensitivity

This is the proportion of those people who really have the disease who are correctly identified as such (TP/TP+FN). For 'sensitivity' to be 100% there must be no false-negative cases. Thus a negative 'sensitivity' test rules out disease.

Specificity

This is the proportion of those subjects who really do not have disease who are correctly identified as such (TN/TN+FP). For 'specificity' to be 100% there must be no false-positive cases. A positive 'specificity' test rules in disease.

3 (i) You have a recent study (Abstract 1) about the accuracy of ultrasound at a 5-mm threshold for abnormality for the detection of endometrial cancer. What are the reported values for:

    (a)   Sensitivity   ----------------- 99% --------------------

    (b)   Specificity   ------------------ 59% -------------------

3 (ii) You have another recent study (Abstract 2) about the accuracy of hysteroscopy for the detection of endometrial cancer.

ABSTRACT 2

Study of: Hysteroscopic evaluation of menopausal patients with sonographic assessment of endometrium.

Aim: To evaluate and compare the diagnostic precision of hysteroscopy in a group of menopausal women in whom D&C was performed.

Methods: A Hamou type II CO_2 hysteroscope was used to evaluate the endocervical canal and the uterine cavity, followed by endometrial sampling.

Results: 39 women were assessed using hysteroscopy and endometrial biopsy. Histopathology results were available for diagnosis in 29 of them (74.3%). In the remaining 10 patients, the hysteroscopic diagnosis was atrophic endometrium. The sensitivity and specificity for hysteroscopy were 53.7% and 96.9%, respectively.

Conclusions: These significant results indicate that this simplified endoscopic method surpasses all blind hospital or office endometrial sampling methods. Therefore, we suggest that hysteroscopy should be the initial assessment tool for any type of indication requiring endometrial and uterine cavity assessment.

What are the reported values for:

(a)   Sensitivity   ------------------ 53.7% --------------------

(b)   Specificity   ----------------- 96.9% ---------------------

3 (iii) Considering the above information, what do you think about the relative diagnostic value of the two tests?

(a) Ultrasound is very suitable for the exclusion (ruling out) of the disease under question (endometrial cancer).

(b) With ultrasound, the probability that the disease under question (*i.e.* cancer) is present despite a negative test result is very low.

(c) Hysteroscopy is very suitable for the exclusion (ruling out) of the disease under question (endometrial cancer).

(d) With hysteroscopy, the probability that the disease under question (*i.e.* cancer) is present despite a negative test result is very low.

A.   All statements (a–d) are incorrect.

B.   The first statement (a) is correct, the second, third and fourth statements (b–d) are incorrect.

C.   The second and third statements (b,c) are correct, the first and fourth statement (a,d) are incorrect.

D.   The first and second statements (a,b) are correct, the third and forth statements (c,d) are incorrect.

E.   All statements (a–d) are correct.

The correct answer is: D

Suggested reading

Clark TJ, Gupta JK. *Handbook of outpatient hysteroscopy: a complete guide to diagnosis and therapy.* London: Hodder Arnold, 2005

Khan KS, Kunz R, Kleijnen J, Antes G. *Systematic reviews to support evidence-based medicine*, 1st edn. London: Royal Society of Medicine Press, 2003.

Mencaglia L, Hamou J. *Manual of Hysteroscopy – Diagnosis and Surgery.* Tuttlingen, Germany: Endo-Press, 2004

Mencaglia L, Hamou E. *Manual of Hysteroscopy – Diagnosis and Surgery.* Tuttlingen, Germany: Endo-Press, 2002.

O'Donovan P *et al. Advances in Gynaecologic Surgery.* London: Greenwich Medical Media, 2001.

Taylor PT, Gordon AG. *Practical Hysteroscopy*, 1st edn. Oxford: Blackwell Scientific Publications, 1993.

Valle R. *Manual of Clinical Hysteroscopy.* London: Taylor and Francis, 2005.

Index

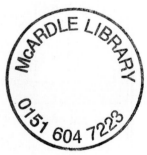

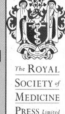
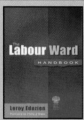
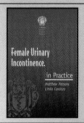
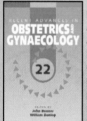
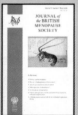